Managing
SUBFERTILITY
in SAFOG Region

Managing
SUBFERTILITY
in SAFOG Region

Editors

Yousaf Latif Khan
MBBS FCPS Dip Endoscopy (France)
Professor, Obstetrics and Gynecology, Rashid Latif Medical College
Lahore, Punjab, Pakistan
Secretary General, SAFOG

Narendra Malhotra
MBBS MD FIAJAGO FICMU FICOG FICMCH FRCOG FICS FMAS AFIAP
Director, International Affairs SAFOG
Managing Director, Global Rainbow Healthcare
Director, ART Rainbow IVF, Agra; Director, MHMH (P) Ltd., Agra
Director, MTTBC, Agra, Uttar Pradesh, India; Director, IAN Donald School
President, INSARAG (2020); Vice President SAFOG (2020) and WAPM (2018)
Past President, ISAR/ISPAT/IFUMB/FOGSI/AOGS/ICMU (Dean)
Founder Editor, SAFOG Journal
Director, SMRITI Manyata CSE
Chairman, SMRITI (NGO)—New Level of Care
President, Rotary Club Agra Taj City

Rohana Haththotuwa
MBBS (SL) MS O&G (Col) FICOG (Hon) FSLCOG FRCOG
Founder Chairman, Ninewells CARE Mother and Baby Hospital, Colombo, Sri Lanka
Secretary General, AOFOG
Immediate Past Chairman, Menstrual Disorders Committee, FIGO
President Elect, South Asian Federation of Obstetrics and Gynaecology (SAFOG)
President, World Gestosis Organization
Past President, Sri Lanka College of Obstetricians and Gynaecologists (SLCOG)
Past President, Menopause Society of Sri Lanka
President Elect, South Asian Federation of Menopause Societies
Treasurer, Asia Pacific Society for Infections in Gynaecology and Obstetrics (2010 till date)
Country Representative, ASPIRE (Asia Pacific Initiative in Reproductive Endocrinology)

Foreword
Gabor Kovacs AM

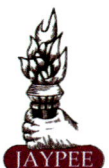

JAYPEE BROTHERS MEDICAL PUBLISHERS
The Health Sciences Publisher
New Delhi | London

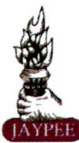 **Jaypee Brothers Medical Publishers (P) Ltd**

Headquarters

Jaypee Brothers Medical Publishers (P) Ltd
EMCA House, 23/23-B
Ansari Road, Daryaganj
New Delhi 110 002, India
Landline: +91-11-23272143, +91-11-23272703
+91-11-23282021, +91-11-23245672
Email: jaypee@jaypeebrothers.com

Corporate Office

Jaypee Brothers Medical Publishers (P) Ltd
4838/24, Ansari Road, Daryaganj
New Delhi 110 002, India
Phone: +91-11-43574357
Fax: +91-11-43574314
Email: jaypee@jaypeebrothers.com

Overseas Office

JP Medical Ltd
83 Victoria Street, London
SW1H 0HW (UK)
Phone: +44 20 3170 8910
Fax: +44 (0)20 3008 6180
Email: info@jpmedpub.com

Website: www.jaypeebrothers.com
Website: www.jaypeedigital.com

© 2022, Jaypee Brothers Medical Publishers

The views and opinions expressed in this book are solely those of the original contributor(s)/author(s) and do not necessarily represent those of editor(s) or publisher of the book.

All rights reserved. No part of this publication may be reproduced, stored or transmitted in any form or by any means, electronic, mechanical, photocopying, recording or otherwise, without the prior permission in writing of the publishers.

All brand names and product names used in this book are trade names, service marks, trademarks or registered trademarks of their respective owners. The publisher is not associated with any product or vendor mentioned in this book.

Medical knowledge and practice change constantly. This book is designed to provide accurate, authoritative information about the subject matter in question. However, readers are advised to check the most current information available on procedures included and check information from the manufacturer of each product to be administered, to verify the recommended dose, formula, method and duration of administration, adverse effects and contraindications. It is the responsibility of the practitioner to take all appropriate safety precautions. Neither the publisher nor the author(s)/editor(s) assume any liability for any injury and/or damage to persons or property arising from or related to use of material in this book.

This book is sold on the understanding that the publisher is not engaged in providing professional medical services. If such advice or services are required, the services of a competent medical professional should be sought.

Every effort has been made where necessary to contact holders of copyright to obtain permission to reproduce copyright material. If any have been inadvertently overlooked, the publisher will be pleased to make the necessary arrangements at the first opportunity. The **CD/DVD-ROM** (if any) provided in the sealed envelope with this book is complimentary and free of cost. **Not meant for sale.**

Inquiries for bulk sales may be solicited at: jaypee@jaypeebrothers.com

Managing Subfertility in SAFOG Region

First Edition: **2022**

ISBN: 978-93-5465-604-0

Printed at: Sterling Graphics Pvt. Ltd.

Dedicated and Pledged to
the health of women in SAFOG countries

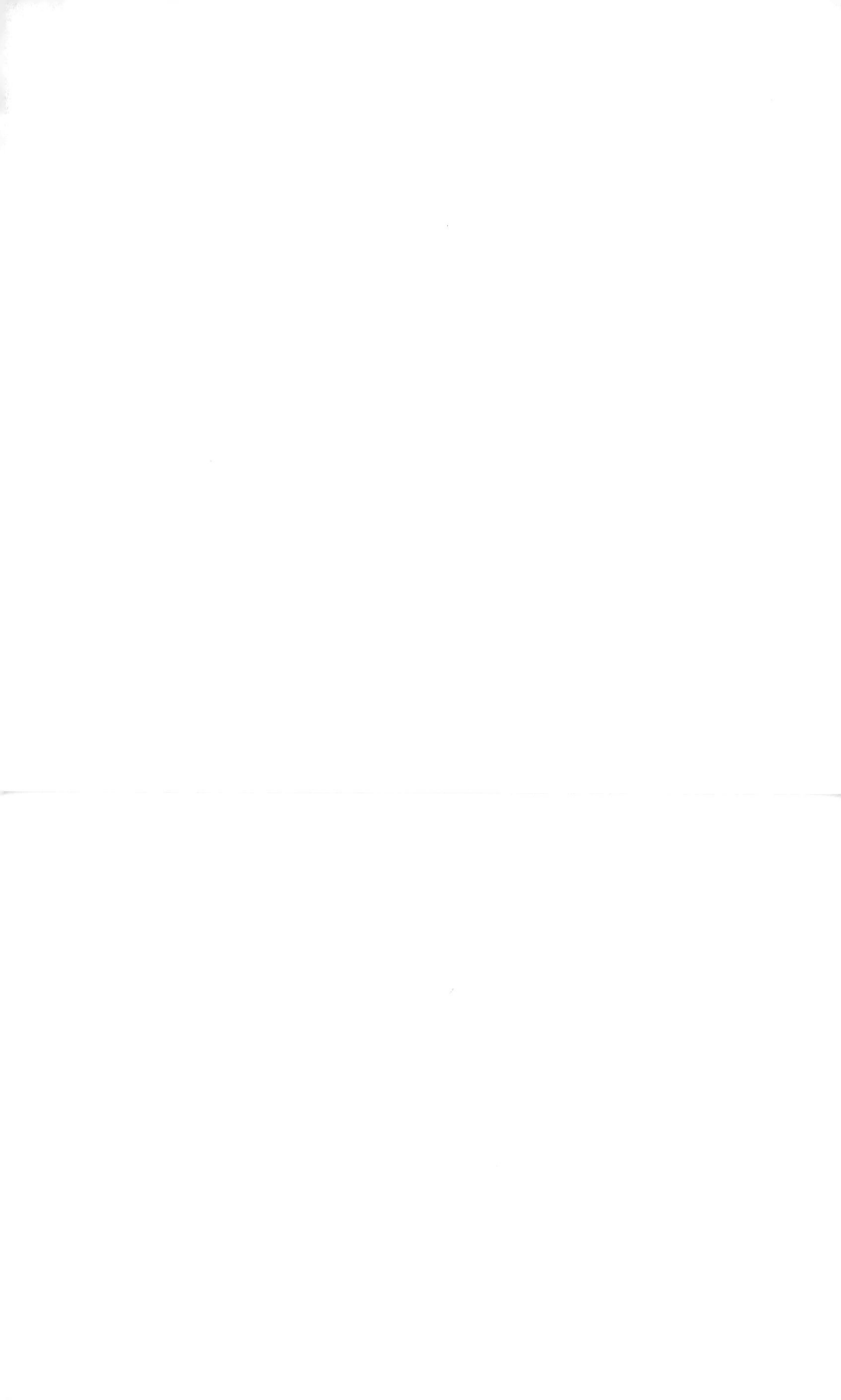

Foreword

Most of the information and research on fertility has traditionally come from Europe or America, but as 60% of the world's population (4.3 billion people) live in Asia-Pacific, it is great to have a book written in Pakistan for the Asia-Pacific community.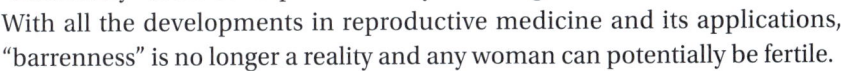

The book is to be commended on using the term "subfertility" as the concept of infertility is no longer valid. With all the developments in reproductive medicine and its applications, "barrenness" is no longer a reality and any woman can potentially be fertile.

The authors are experienced gynecologists, who have provided the A to Z of fertility treatment. This is a very comprehensive review of all the possible investigations and treatments that a couple with subfertility would have suggested to them, and enables these consumers to get all the information they need to expand on what is covered in the medical consultation.

The book commences with a thorough and easily understandable description of both male and female anatomy and physiology, which all readers need to understand. They then explain the physiology of how pregnancy occurs, before launching into the area of subfertility.

There is an extensive list of the possible causes of difficulty to conceive, both male and female, before describing the investigations that can be carried out.

The book then concentrates on the possible treatments that may be considered, as well as general advice about personal health such as weight control and avoidance of smoking.

The book also describes the value of counseling including explanation and reassurance.

The second half of the book is devoted to a detailed description of available treatments.

The authors are to be commended on a very readable but detailed description of available treatments. A whole chapter is devoted to assisted reproductive technique (ART) which is probably the most important and widely used treatment in 2021, with detailed description of each of the steps involved.

The authors have also devoted a chapter to practices that are not practiced in all clinics because of religious or moral objections, but are carried out in others, such as sperm and egg donation and surrogacy, so it is important to include these for a complete reference.

The book is concluded by a chapter on adoption and accepting childlessness which is helpful to the minority of couples who do not proceed with treatment, or do not succeed.

I believe that this book would be a very worthwhile read for all couples with difficulty conceiving, it is easy to read, and can be understood by the lay people without extensive medical knowledge, as well as introductory reading for medical, nursing and scientific staff commencing work in this area.

Gabor Kovacs AM
MBBS HONS MD FRCOG FRANZCOG CREI Grad Dip Mgt (Macq)
Professor of Obstetrics and Gynecology
Monash University
Melbourne, Australia
Editor-in-Chief, Fertility and Reproduction

Preface

Subfertility: Failure to achieve a pregnancy
- 80% couples have pregnancy within 2 years
- 15–20% need treatment

Generally, speaking even if a healthy couple does not practice contraception *it may take up to 1 year to conceive*. Even after a year of regular coitus (2–3 times a week) without contraception, there is only 70–80% chance of conception. Those couples who live separately due to social and professional reasons, and do not have regular and frequent coitus may take longer to conceive. *In couples where the wife is above 35 years, coitus is infrequent (only over the weekend) and if there is some abnormality, it may take longer than even 2 years for the couple to conceive.*

There is 15–20% probability of a married couple seeking advice for their involuntary subfertility. Couples who have this problem face heavy social, psychological, and family pressure. They suffer from great disappointment, anguish, frustration, and depression. Every month they hope and pray for pregnancy but with the onset of menstruation their hopes are shattered. However, they never give up, and keep trying and hoping each month.

In South Asian countries, cultural norm is to expect the bride to become pregnant within the first few months of marriage. If she does not become pregnant within 4–6 months the family in general, and mother-in-law in particular, gets anxious. The family start worrying, without realizing that it may be a planned action on the part of the couple. The whole family starts pressurizing the couple to seek medical advice.

For such couples, there is now genuine and real hope. These couples are living in an era where most of them can be successfully treated. The latest technology can be useful in the treatment of most of the factors responsible for their subfertility. Unfortunately, a large number of these couples are unaware of the available help. This may be due to a lack of knowledge about the physiology of the reproductive system or due to a lack of information about the methods of assistance available.

Finally a word of caution. Although it may seem that a cure is possible in every case and therefore the rate of successful treatment should be nearly 100%. It is unfortunately not so. Nature has many secrets which, we have not been able to unfold as yet. This explains why a large number of couples suffer from *unexplained subfertility*. For such couples all the investigations remain negative and no one can pinpoint the causative factors. There are bound to be a few disappointments. We should accept this as God's will and hope that in the near future new breakthroughs will make their treatment possible.

Preface

We hope the readers find this book informative enough and also hope that after reading this book, the readers' perception about your possible problems and their treatment is clearer.

We wish you good luck.

Yousaf Latif Khan
Narendra Malhotra
Rohana Haththotuwa

Editors Note

This book is intended to acquaint subfertile couples with and young practitioners with the basic functioning and the mechanism of the human reproductive system. It has been written in simple language so that the readers can understand the problem and appreciate possible remedies. To some of the readers this book may seem too simple and brief. For those interested in advanced reading, advanced medical books can be consulted. On the other hand, some may find it too technical for lay persons. *In that case we would suggest skipping first four chapters and straight away to go on to investigations of subfertility.*

Yousaf Latif Khan
Narendra Malhotra
Rohana Haththotuwa

Contents

1. Why Pregnancy 1
2. Anatomy and Physiology 3
3. How Pregnancy Takes Place? 10
4. Causes of Subfertility 16
5. Investigations of Subfertility 21
6. Treatment of Subfertility (Female Factors) 32
7. Assisted Reproductive Techniques (Test Tube Baby) 43
8. Treatment of Subfertility (Male Factors) 51
9. Donor Egg/Sperm and Surrogacy 55
10. How to Prepare for a Pregnancy? 58
11. Acceptance of Childlessness and Adoption 67
12. Normal Laboratory Values 71

Glossary 77

Index 87

CHAPTER 1

Why Pregnancy?

■ INTRODUCTION

God created the universe and blessed all living things with the ability to procreate. This is God's greatest gift to all living beings. Ever since the evolution of society began, the human beings have been extremely conscious of this fact. To be the master of the world, man had to outnumber so many large and powerful, but less intelligent, animals.

Numerical superiority is the basic necessity for maintaining control over this planet. May be the purpose of life itself is not fulfilled without procreation. The instinctive desire to reproduce has to be satisfied. There could also be a desire for reproduction for inheritance of name and property. It could simply be pressure from senior members of the family or a mother-in-law, who want a couple to have a baby immediately after their marriage, contrary to what the couple desires about starting a family.

It is common to meet couples not having any desire to reproduce. If anything, they are averse to this idea. In such couples, lack of interest in one partner will be frustrating the desire of the other by being noncooperative. This noncooperation may manifest in infrequent coitus or reluctance to have proper guidance and investigations. This negative attitude is usually due to personal reasons but it could also be due to a conviction that any further additions to an already overpopulated world would be detrimental. The couple may feel that they would be unable to look after the child as well as they would wish. This may be due to economic, social, or professional reasons. However, such couples are in a minority. Most of the couples do wish to have at least one baby; in some cases at least one male.

Yet, unfortunately, in every society there is a large percentage of couples who are unable to produce a baby. In spite of their best efforts and application, they fail to procreate. They fail to achieve what comes naturally and in abundance to others. They try desperately every month without any luck. One can imagine their disappointment and desperation.

Unfortunately, 20% of all the married couples suffer from involuntary subfertility which leads to frustration and unhappiness. These subfertile couples welcome, and in fact, seek any kind of help, assistance or treatment which is forthcoming. Therefore, it is quite common to see even educated couples being duped, swindled and mismanaged by quacks. They also frequent shrines to make offerings/sacrifices in the name of *Peers/Fakirs*.

2 Why Pregnancy?

Whatever is the motive or driving force for such a desperate desire to have a baby, it is important that the problem should be clearly comprehended and scientifically/professionally treated. Instead of running from pillar to post and knocking at the doors of imposters, charlatans and cheats, such couples must know the causes of subfertility and available remedies. To save such couples from this fruitless yet expensive exercise, I have written the following chapters. I do hope they fulfill the objective.

CHAPTER 2

Anatomy and Physiology

■ INTRODUCTION

This chapter gives a brief description of the structure and function of the organs which play a vital role in reproduction or pregnancy.

We have tried to keep it simple. If you feel it is too elaborate, or too technical, you can skip this and move on to the next chapter.

The organs involved in reproduction are known as the *genital organs*, they are present in males as well as females. These organs are divided into:
- *External*: They lie on surface of the body and are visible.
- *Internal*: They lie inside the body and are not visible.

■ MALE EXTERNAL GENITAL ORGANS (FIG. 1)

These organs lie on the surface of the body and are either visible to the eye or can be felt by physical examination.

The following are the external male genital organs:
- Penis (male organ, phallus)
- Scrotum
- Testes
- Ducts

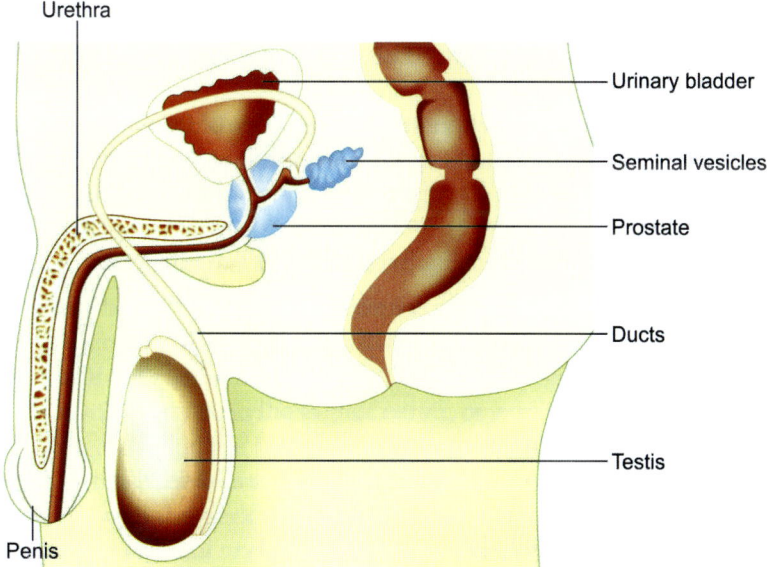

Fig. 1: Male genital organs.

Penis

This is the main organ of reproduction in a male. Normally it is in a flaccid form and hangs between and front of thighs. Through its roots, it is attached to the pelvic bones. The penis has a body or shaft and its end is known as the glans. The tip or glans is normally covered by a fold of loose skin which is excised during circumcision. The last part of urinary tract (urethra) runs through the shaft of the penis and opens at its end. The urethra is used as a passage for urination and for the passage of semen during ejaculation.

The urethra in the penis is surrounded by erectile tissue. This erectile tissue is like a sponge with many empty spaces in it. When these spaces get filled up with blood, erection takes place. During erection the shaft becomes rigid, stands on its roots, and it increases in length and breadth.

The size of the penis may vary, depending on the state it is in. In a flaccid state, its length varies from 5 to 11 cm, and in an erect state from 14 to 19 cm. The size is neither related to height or weight of a man nor to the length in a flaccid condition. The size has no relationship with the capacity of fertility either.

Misconceptions like the penis being too small or the tilt in the flaccid form are common among some men. They need to know that the size in the flaccid form in no way affects reproduction. As long as the penis can penetrate into the vagina and deposit semen inside, it is good enough for reproduction. The tilt of the penis in flaccid position of the penis is not a defect and there is no need to worry about it.

Scrotum

This is a bag of skin which hangs from the root of the penis, between the upper parts of thighs. It has two compartments and within each compartment lies a testis.

Nature has made the scrotum to keep the testes outside the abdomen. The purpose is to keep the testes cool, because the temperature inside the abdomen is high, whereas the temperature in the scrotum is slightly below the body temperature. This keeps the temperature of the testes at a lower level. It is important because if the testes are kept at a high temperature (inside the abdomen or hot baths) the sperm production is either reduced (oligospermia) or may stop (azoospermia).

Sometimes the accumulation of fluid inside the scrotum (hydrocele) or dilated veins (varicocele) may be present. In such conditions, production of sperm is affected and the man may suffer from reduced sperm motility or sperm count.

Testes (Male Gonads)

There are two testes which lie in each compartment of the scrotum.

The testes perform two functions:
1. Production of sperms (spermatozoa, germ cells)
2. Production of secretions (hormones, testosterone)

The testes produce millions of sperms. They are released from the testes into a narrow duct or passage. They take 75 days to mature and travel up the ducts. Through these ducts the sperms reach the urethra where they are joined by the secretions of the prostate gland and seminal vesicles. These secretions are essential for their motility and capacity to penetrate the female egg. In the absence of these secretions, the sperms lack the ability to fertilize the female egg.

The sperms are important for the fertilization of the female egg (pregnancy). The male hormone (testosterone) is essential for the growth of the male features, beard, hair, and masculine growth especially the growth of the sexual organs. Testosterone also influences the desire for sex (libido).

The male hormone (testosterone) gets into the blood straight from the testes. Through the bloodstream, the hormone reaches the areas or organs where it is required to act.

Ducts (Vas Deferens)

These ducts are long and narrow which conduct the male germ cells from the testes to the urethra. The ends of these ducts near the testes are dilated and broad. From testes, sperms enter into the dilated part of ducts (epididymis) through many narrow tubes. From each testis, duct travels upward into the abdomen. It passes through the groin and can be felt as a thin but firm cord in the groin. Just before the duct enters the urethra in the prostate gland, it is joined by the seminal vesicles.

■ MALE INTERNAL GENITAL ORGANS

Seminal Vesicles

The seminal vesicles are a pair of small tubes which are located at the base of the bladder near the prostate gland. These tubes also join the urethra inside the prostate gland; they are also joined by ducts from the testes. They act as storage for sperms which are continuously produced by the testes. The seminal vesicles produce secretions which along with the secretions of the prostate gland and the bulbourethral glands help to improve the movement (motility) of the spermatozoa. The semen discharged during one coitus (ejaculate) contains millions of sperms, secretions from seminal vesicles, and other glands.

Prostate Gland

This gland is located at base of the bladder. It is normally the size of a walnut (2–2.50 cm). The structure of this gland is like a sponge and it has a few

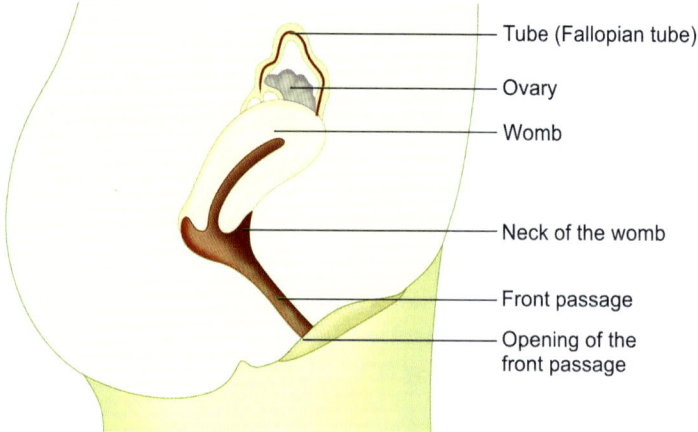

Fig. 2: Female genital organs (side view).

muscle fibers. The gland has many small ducts which open into the urethra during its passage through this gland. The urethra leaves the base of the bladder and passes through the prostate gland.

■ FEMALE EXTERNAL GENITAL ORGANS (FIG. 2)

The organs are collectively known as vulva. The vulva is not as important as the male external genital organs. It is located around the opening of the female front passage (introitus). Bartholin's glands in the vulva are located at this opening. The glands are two in number and are of small size, the size of a pea.

The glands produce watery secretions during sexual intercourse (coitus). The small urethral opening for the passage of urine is located just above the opening of the female front passage. The opening of the intestinal tract (anus) is located 1–2 inches behind opening of the front passage.

■ FEMALE INTERNAL GENITAL ORGANS AND GONADS (FIG. 3)

The female internal genital organs are as follows. They are listed from below upward:
- Female front passage (vagina)
- Womb (uterus)
- Tubes (Fallopian tubes)
- Ovaries (female gonads)

Front Passage (Vagina)

This is the lowest part of the female internal genital organs. This is a thin walled, muscular, hollow, stretchable tube. It lies between the terminal parts of the urinary and intestinal tracts.

Anatomy and Physiology

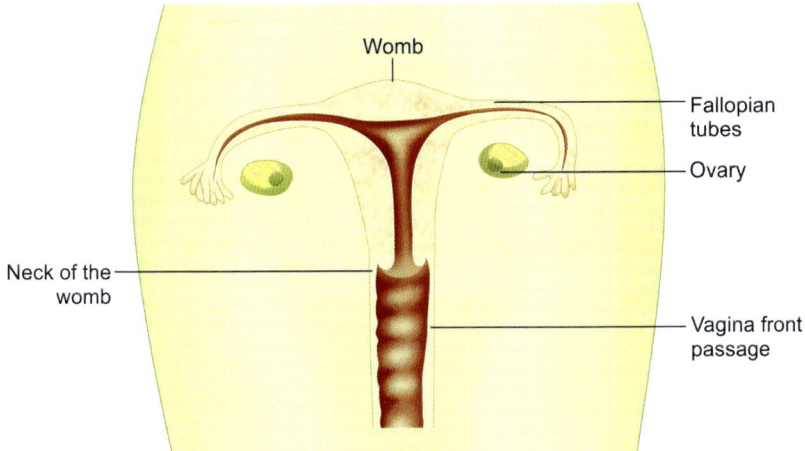

Fig. 3: Female genital organs (front view).

The lower end of the front passage is at the vulva. At its upper end the cervix projects into it. In virgins, the lower end of the front passage has a thin membrane, known as the *hymen*. The hymen usually gets torn during the first sexual intercourse.

Normally, the front passage is kept closed with the front and back walls lie touching each other. Due to its ability to stretch it opens up during sexual intercourse (coitus) and child birth.

The front passage is normally kept moist by small and clear secretions which are colorless and odorless. These secretions, when produced in excess, come out from the front passage and may stain underclothes (leukorrhea). Extra production of these secretions takes place during sexual excitement and sometimes without sexual excitement. A girl may complain of *"white vaginal discharge"*. This discharge is colorless, odorless, and nonirritating. It needs no treatment except explanation and reassurance. But if it is profuse, yellowish or having an odor and irritating, it will need treatment.

Womb (Uterus)

This is a hollow, muscular pear-shaped organ with thick walls. The pear lies upside down with its tip (cervix) projecting into the top end of the front passage (vagina).

In a normal womb, the thickness of the walls is 1.5 cm and the cavity is small, like a slit. The cavity of the womb communicates at its lower end with the front passage and at its upper end with the lumen of the two tubes.

The lining of the womb (endometrium) changes its thickness in response to secretions (hormones) produced by the ovaries. During childbearing age, thickness of the lining of the cavity, gradually increases every month (in a cyclical fashion). The duration of the cycle is usually of 22–35 days. At the end of the cycle this lining is shed. The shed lining comes out through the front passage in the form of "periods" or menstruation; and lasts for 2–8 days. The amount of normal blood loss, every month, is about 80–100 mL. If pregnancy takes place during any cycle, then shedding does not take place and there is no menstrual bleeding at the end of that cycle.

Tubes (Fallopian Tubes)

These are two hollow tubes which are narrow, long, and muscular. Each tube is attached to one side of the upper end of the womb.

They have an opening at the outer end (fimbrial end). Through this opening the lumen of the tube communicates with the abdominal cavity. The ovaries lie close to this opening. The other end of the tube communicates with the cavity of the womb.

The female egg which is produced by one of the ovaries (ovulation) enters the fallopian tube immediately after its release. In the outer part of the fallopian tube, it meets the sperms which reach that part of the tube with movements of their own tail. Millions of spermatozoa reach the egg and surround it but only one enters the egg and causes pregnancy (fertilization). The rest of the sperms are also essential to facilitate entry of one spermatozoon into the egg.

For a pregnancy, at least one of these tubes should be open. If both tubes are blocked, then spontaneous pregnancy cannot take place. The passage of the female egg through the tubes is helped by special lining cells of lumen of the tube and by muscular wall movements, which push the egg into the cavity of the womb.

Ovaries (Female Gonads)

The ovaries which are female equivalent of the male testes are two in number and lie in the pelvis near outer ends of the fallopian tubes.

The ovaries are almond shaped, solid, grayish white structures. Their measurements are approximately 3.0 cm × 2.5 cm × 1.0 cm. Their surface contains a large number of follicles (primitive eggs). The ovaries are nonfunctioning before the age of 12–13 years (puberty) and after the age of 45–50 years (menopause).

Between the ages of 12 and 50 years, ovaries perform two functions:
1. Production of female eggs (ovum)
2. Production of female hormones (estrogens and progesterone)

These two activities are performed in a cyclical fashion. This cycle is usually of 28–30 days.

Soon after puberty and a few years before the onset of menopause (around 50 years of age) the cycle may become erratic or irregular.

The ovaries produce female egg, usually in the middle of the cycle, and female hormones are produced throughout the cycle. The hormones are of two types: (1) estrogens and (2) progesterone. Estrogens are produced throughout the cycle. Progesterone is produced only after release of female egg on the 14th or 15th days of the cycle, i.e., during latter half of the cycle. The presence of progesterone in the second half of the cycle is an indication that ovulation has taken place.

These hormones are essential for the female growth of the body, especially for the growth of female genital organs, breasts, and maintenance of pregnancy.

God has been extra kind to all the species. He has given us all the essential organs in pairs. There are two eyes, two ears, two lungs, two kidneys, two ovaries, two testes, and two tubes. Although only one of these organs is good enough to perform its functions but He has provided a reserve, in case one organ is damaged the other will take over its functions.

Provided the ovary and the tube are healthy, pregnancy can take place with only one ovary and one fallopian tube. In case of damage or removal of one tube or ovary, the chances of pregnancy are the same as in any other woman.

CHAPTER 3

How Pregnancy Takes Place?

■ INTRODUCTION

In the preceding chapter, anatomy of the male and female genital organs has been described. It tells us the site of production of sperms (spermatozoa) and the female egg cell (ovum). It also tells us about the narrow passages through which male sperms and the female egg travel for their union. *This union of male sperms and female egg is called fertilization of egg which is the beginning of a pregnancy* (**Flowchart 1**).

In order to understand the mechanism of fertilization, this chapter is divided into the following sections:

- Sperms (spermatozoa, male germ cells)
- Male sex hormones
- Female eggs (ovum, "ova" plural)
- Sexual intercourse (coitus)
- Pregnancy (fertilization of the egg)
- Implantation (embedding of the fertilized egg)
- Sex of the baby (fetus).

Flowchart 1: How pregnancy takes place?

```
                    Fertility (pregnancy)
                   /                     \
              Husband                    Wife
                 │                        │
              Sperms                     Eggs
                 │                        │
          Ability for coitus           Open tubes
                 │
        Release of sperms
            in vagina
                 │
        Movement of sperms
           to reach egg
                 │                        │
                 └──→ Union of sperms ←──┘
                         and egg
                            │
                        Pregnancy
```

■ SPERMS (SPERMATOZOA, MALE GERM CELLS)

The sperms provide the male part for a pregnancy (fertilization of the egg). They are produced in millions in the testes of an adult male. Their production is almost continuous in both the testes. The sperms are tiny motile (moving) cells which can be seen only with the help of a microscope. These cells have a head and a tail. The whipping movement of their tails enables the sperms to move forward very fast.

During sexual intercourse, the sperms are deposited in the upper part of the vagina. The male sperms move fast toward the egg through the vagina to the womb and finally reach the outer part of the fallopian tubes where the ovum (egg) lies. In this part, the union of one spermatozoa and one egg takes place. This is how fertilization or pregnancy is achieved.

If for some reason, the sperms are not motile and cannot reach the female egg, pregnancy will not take place.

The number of chromosomes in a normal human cell is 46. All cells in the body have the same fixed number of chromosomes. The sperm and the female egg carry only half the number of chromosomes as that of a normal human cell (23). Each egg carries one sex chromosome named X. The sex chromosomes in case of sperms are of two types, X and Y chromosomes (all female eggs carry the same sex chromosome called X). During fertilization chromosomes from an egg is the same irrespective of the sex of the baby. On the other hand, half of sperms carry X chromosome and other half carry Y chromosome. The egg may be fertilized by sperm carrying X or Y chromosome.

Although there are millions of sperms yet only one sperm is required for pregnancy (fertilization). Out of millions of sperms only one succeeds in fertilizing the egg. There is an equal chance that the fertilizing sperm may carry an X chromosome or Y chromosome.

If pregnancy takes place with the sperm carrying the X chromosome, then the sex of the baby is female and if the fertilizing sperm carries a Y chromosome, then the sex of the baby is male. *The sex of the baby is purely decided by the type of sperm causing pregnancy, and is determined at the time of fertilization. It cannot change later on.*

■ MALE SEX HORMONES

The production of sperms is controlled by hormones produced in the body.

Although all body hormones have some influence on the production of sperms, the following hormones play a major role in the control of their production:
- Gonadotropic hormones [follicle-stimulating hormone (FSH) and luteinizing hormone (LH)] produced by a small gland located at the base of the brain, called the pituitary gland. They stimulate testes to produce sperms and testosterone hormone.

- *Testosterone hormone*: This is the male hormone produced in the testes by Leydig cells. These cells lie outside the tubules where the sperms are produced. Leydig cells are more stable than sperms. Due to this factor, heat or infection destroys the sperms but Leydig cells continue to produce the hormone (testosterone). This hormone plays an important role in the growth of the secondary sexual characters and other masculine features such as deepening of voice and growth of the body.

    The level of testosterone may influence the desire for sex (virility) but does not, generally, influence the chances of fertility.

    In addition to these hormones, production of sperms is also influenced by general health, acute or chronic infections, stress (psychological and physical), diet, climate, metabolic disease (diabetes, jaundice, etc.) and local diseases. Smoking and alcohol, especially in excess, have an adverse effect on their production.

■ FEMALE EGG (OVUM, PLURAL "OVA")

The female eggs are produced in the ovaries. During childbearing age, only one egg is produced during one ovarian cycle in a month. This egg is produced either by the right or left ovary. The egg is a large cell, and like sperms contains half the number of chromosomes (23).

The female egg gradually matures in the ovary. It is usually released from the ovary in the middle of the menstrual cycle. Once it is released from the ovary, the egg is sucked into the fallopian tube through its opening. The egg stays in the lumen of the tube. If it is not fertilized within 24 hours, the egg degenerates and dies away. It means that if pregnancy does not take place within 24 hours of release of the egg from the ovary the egg dies and degenerates. The chance of becoming pregnant is stronger only in the middle of the ovarian cycle and that too only within 24 hours or so upon the release of the egg.

The ripening and release of the egg (maturation and ovulation) are under the control of various hormones. These hormones are produced by the pituitary gland located at the base of the brain. This gland produces FSH and LH hormones. The production of FSH and LH is controlled by the brain and is also influenced by estrogens and progesterone. Every month at the beginning of the cycle, under the influence of hormones, one of the eggs starts ripening in its follicle and by the middle of the cycle (approximately 12–14 days after start of the cycle) the egg is released from its follicle (ovulation). During this period, only estrogens are produced from follicles in the ovary. After the release of the egg the follicle is called corpus luteum, and it produces female hormones (estrogens and progesterone) which are essential for maintenance of a pregnancy. If the fertilization of an egg does not take place, then at end of the cycle (usually duration of the cycle is 28 days) the lining of the womb undergoes degeneration which appears in the form of menstrual blood (periods).

■ SEXUAL INTERCOURSE (COITUS)

Sexual intercourse means penetration of the penis into the front passage (vagina) of a female. This act is also called "sex" or "coitus".

The valves in the veins of the penis which drain blood out of it normally do not obstruct blood flowing out of it. During sexual excitement these valves block veins with the result that outflow of blood is blocked and inflow continues through the arteries. The blood accumulates in the spongy tissues of the penis causing accumulation of blood. The penis increases in length and width, it also becomes firm and erect.

During sexual excitement the secretions of seminal vesicles, sperms, and prostate secretions are poured into this part of the urethra. These secretions pass through the urethra as an ejaculate (man's discharge during intercourse). This discharge is a milky white, thick fluid with a special odor. Its volume is 1.5–3.0 mL.

During this act, the semen is usually deposited by the male partner, high up in the front passage. Nature has provided us with a desire for this act and also has made it enjoyable for the purposes of reproduction. The desire for this act is spontaneous and usually the other partner is initiated into it by preliminary kissing, hugging, and tender handling.

The frequency of this act varies, but in most married couples coitus takes place usually 2–3 times a week. The desire of this physical act is influenced by social, psychological, and physical factors. The psychological factors (stress, anxiety, depression, etc.) are the most common causes of inability to perform this act (*impotency or frigidity*). Physical factors are less common.

Physiologically, sexual intercourse is controlled by the nervous system (brain), hormonal system, and physical well-being of a man. The desire for sex and the act of sex are influenced by the presence of hormones in the body. A male partner reaches orgasm in most cases but the duration of the act is extremely variable. It can last for less than a minute or it may be prolonged for a longer period (5–15 minutes).

The female partner may not always achieve an orgasm, and at times, may not participate enthusiastically in the act. The *absence of an orgasm and lack of interest in the act has no direct relationship to her ability to reproduce.*

Lastly, it may be added that an orgasm makes the sexual intercourse enjoyable between partners but has no relationship with the chances of a pregnancy. The production of egg and healthy sperms has no direct relationship to coitus and production of hormones.

■ FERTILIZATION

The spermatozoa are active (motile), due to the movement of their tail, run upward through the vagina, mouth of the womb (cervix) into the cavity of the womb, and then into the fallopian tubes of the uterus, where these spermatozoa meet the female egg. One of these sperms enters the egg and causes fertilization. This is how a pregnancy takes place.

Once semen is placed inside the vagina, the sperms are capable of fertilization of the egg even after 4–5 days. On the other hand, once the egg is released, from the ovary, it can only survive for up to 24 hours. If it is not fertilized within 24 hours, it undergoes degeneration and pregnancy cannot take place. During each month, only one egg is released from the ovary.

Once the fertilized egg reaches cavity of the womb, it remains there for 9 months and grows into a fully mature baby.

▋ ESTABLISHMENT OF PREGNANCY (IMPLANTATION)

When the union of sperm and female egg takes place, the number of chromosomes in the fertilized egg is complete. It is as many as those in a normal cell (46). Secondly, the sex of the baby (fetus) is determined at this stage. It depends upon which type of sperm has caused the pregnancy. If a sperm carrying an X chromosome is responsible for fertilization, then sex of the baby will be a female. On the other hand, if the sperm responsible for fertilization of the egg is carrying a Y chromosome, then the sex of the baby will be a male. The sex of a baby is decided at the time of fertilization. *No prayer or treatment can change this subsequently.*

After fertilization, the egg spends approximately 3–4 days in the tube (fallopian tube). The fertilized egg gradually moves toward the cavity of the womb and reaches it on the 4th or 5th day. During this period, this egg gets its nourishment from secretions present in the lumen of the tube.

The egg does not move on its own. It is pushed toward the cavity of the womb by movements of the muscular wall of the fallopian tubes (peristalsis) and wave-like movements of projections from lining cells of the fallopian tubes (cilia).

The egg starts dividing soon after fertilization. The first division takes place within 24 hours but subsequent divisions appear at shorter intervals. The egg divides first into two cells then four, eight, and sixteen cells. The fertilized egg is called an *embryo* and subsequently develops into fetus, placenta, and membranes of the pregnancy.

The lining of the cavity of the womb which is already prepared for the reception of this early embryo, provides it with early nourishment from secretions produced by its glands. The embryo lives on these secretions for 2–3 days. By the 6th or 7th day, the embryo develops a layer (trophoblast) which invades the lining of the cavity and produces hormones. The trophoblast penetrates deep into lining of the womb causing local bleeding initially but later development of placenta takes place at this site. The placenta or afterbirth supplies all nourishment to the growing baby inside the womb during the rest of its stay in this cavity (9 months).

The baby, afterbirth, and covering membranes, all develop from the fertilized egg. They all come out at the time of delivery.

■ SEX OF THE BABY

As discussed earlier, the sex of the baby is decided at the time of the union of sperm and female egg. *The sex is determined purely by the sperm.* The female egg does not play any part in this vital decision-making.

Every time a pregnancy takes place, there are 50% chances of it being a male or female baby. If we look at a larger population, this ratio is generally maintained in nature. But if we look at a smaller population (families or groups), one may feel the dominance of males or females in a group or a family. This is purely a chance happening.

CHAPTER 4

Causes of Subfertility

■ INTRODUCTION

Subfertility means the inability of a couple to conceive. In case of a woman, it is the inability to become pregnant; and in case of a man, it is the inability to make a woman pregnant. A healthy couple takes an average of 1 year to achieve a pregnancy. If a couple fails to conceive after 2 years of regular sexual intercourse without contraception (2–3 times/week), they are considered to be subfertile. Statistically, among subfertile couples, 30% are due to a problem with the husband, and 30% are due to a problem with the wife, another 30% due to a problem with both partners, and 10% are unexplained. In some couples even after detailed investigations one may fail to pinpoint a reason for failure to conceive. These couples are considered as a case of *unexplained subfertility*.

There are various causes of subfertility. The cause could be in the male partner or the female partner, or the defect may be in both.

■ CAUSES OF SUBFERTILITY IN MALE PARTNER

The defect could be due to an inadequate production of sperms (male germ cells, spermatozoa) or in the conducting tubes (vas deferens). Sometimes it is due to the inability of the man to perform sexual intercourse (impotency).

The following are likely defects in male partner:
- Defect in production of sperms (spermatogenesis)
- Obstruction in the passages (vas deferens)
- Failure to deposit semen in the front passage (vagina).

Defect in Production of Sperms (Spermatogenesis)

The defect in testes may be so gross that sperms are not produced at all. In such cases the semen does not have any sperms. Doctors call it azoospermia.

On the other hand, defects may be that sperms produced are either in small numbers (oligospermia), or defective in their movements (asthenospermia) or in their form (morphology).

The common causes are:
- *Chromosomal defects*: In such cases, either the testes are not developed or they are underdeveloped. Usually such cases have azoospermia. The common chromosomal defect seen in males is that, men are tall, but eunuchoid type. They have one extra female chromosome (47, XXY) (Klinefelter syndrome).

- *Undescended testes*: The testes fail to descend. In the early stages of the development of a male child inside the womb of the mother, the testes are located inside his abdomen. Gradually they move downward and eventually, come out of the abdomen to lie inside the scrotum. *This descent is essential for the production of sperms*. If for any reason, testes do not descend out of the abdomen due to the heat inside, they do not produce sperms but they can still produce male hormones. In such males, they have all the masculine features, but no sperms in their semen. It is detected at birth that the child has undescended testes and if this defect is corrected during early childhood (1–2 years), then production of sperms may initiate. If this operation is performed later in life, then damage is permanent. The production of sperms will not initiate after late surgery and it will not help fertility, but may save the man from development of serious complications later in life (cancer of testes).
- *Damage to testes*: The testes may be damaged due to the following:
  - *Injury or accidents*: Direct trauma to testes may cause functional damage.
  - *Infection*: In 20–40% cases, *mumps* can cause an infection of the testes, thereby causing permanent damage. It shows importance of vaccination in newborn babies as a preventive measure.
  - Tuberculosis and syphilis can sometimes damage testes.
  - *Surgery*: Any operation on testes, scrotum, or groin can cause damage to the testes. Since the blood supply to the testes is through the groin, it is important that during an operation for hernia the surgeon must ensure that the blood supply to the testes is not compromised. A reduced blood supply can damage the testes.
  - *X-rays*: Prolonged exposure to irradiation (accidentally or for treatment), suppresses sperm production.
  - *Chemotherapy*: The drugs used for chemotherapy for cancer are very toxic to the testes. They usually damage sperm production in the testes. Those men who need chemotherapy, and have a desire to conserve their fertility, need to deposit a large number of spermatozoa in the *cryopreservation bank* (special deep freezer, with very low temperatures). Cryopreservation can save sperms for many years. When there is need, these sperms can be brought out, thawed and used for fertility purposes, usually in in vitro fertilization (IVF), intracytoplasmic sperm injection (ICSI) (test tube baby).
  - Tumors of the testes can cause damage to sperm production in testes.
  - *Suppression of sperm production in healthy testes*: Sperm production may be suppressed under the following circumstances:
    - Local diseases of scrotum (*hydrocele, varicocele*)
    - Hot climate and repeated hot baths
    - Any acute or chronic illness

- Drugs, especially anticancer drugs
- Other hormonal defects in the body
- Excessive smoking and drinking of alcohol
- Deficiency of essential nutritional elements
- Toxic environment.

Obstruction in the Passages

Obstruction in the tubes (vas deferens) on both sides causes absence of sperms in the semen (azoospermia).

The causes of obstruction are:
- *Congenital*: During development of the child in mother's womb the tubes develop defectively and remain closed.
- *Infections*: Gonococcal infection of the tubes cause blockage on both sides. Sometimes *tuberculosis* or other infections may cause blockage of both tubes.
- *Surgery*: Injury to the tube during repair of hernia in the groin may cause blockage. But blockage of one tube does not cause azoospermia whereas blockage of both tubes, as during vasectomy (operation for family planning), will cause azoospermia.

Failure to Deposit Semen in Vagina

- *Impotence*: The impotency may be temporary or permanent and it may be only for a particular partner. The most common cause of impotency is *psychological*, other causes are uncommon.
- *Malformation of penis*: Particularly in hypospadias, semen is deposited outside the female front passage.
- Noncooperation of female partner (vaginismus).

■ CAUSES OF SUBFERTILITY IN FEMALE PARTNER

Following are the causes of subfertility in female partner:
- Defect in production of female egg (ovulation)
- Obstruction in the passage
- Hostility of passage to husband's spermatozoa.

Defect in Production of Female Egg (Ovulation)

In the absence of the female egg, pregnancy cannot take place.

Absence of menstruation: Amenorrhea (absence of menstruation) in most of the cases is associated with absence of production of egg. Nevertheless, all cases of absence of menstruation may not include failure of production of egg. It is common to see pregnancy during absence of menses due to breastfeeding (lactation).

Those women who have either menstrual irregularity or absence of menstruation (amenorrhea) are likely cases of either infrequent ovulation or absence of ovulation. Those who are overweight or grossly underweight are likely to have infrequent ovulation. Sometimes patients take hormonal treatment to regulate their menstrual cycles. Most of these hormonal preparations suppress ovulation. They may regulate menstrual cycles but in the process they inadvertently may be suppressing their ovulation which could be the cause of subfertility.

Obstruction in the Passages

The site of obstruction is mostly in the female tubes. When both tubes are blocked, subfertility occurs. Congenital absence of vagina creates obstruction to the menstrual flow which leads to absence of menstruation and subfertility. In a case of absent uterus, there will be amenorrhea and subfertility.

The common causes of tubal obstruction are as follows:
- *Infection*: Tuberculosis, gonococcal, chlamydial or infection following abortion or after child birth may cause blockage of the female tubes on both sides.
- *Sexually transmitted infections (STI)*: Gonococcal, chlamydia, and bacterial vaginosis (BV).
- *Endometriosis*: This is the condition in which lining of the womb is misplaced and it is present outside the cavity of the womb. It causes multiple problems in women and one of them is subfertility. The mechanism by which the patients with endometriosis and subfertile is not known with clarity but it is presumed that in these patients there is infrequent production of egg and also some interference with the functions of the tubes. Most of the patients suffer from subfertility but they can be helped by modern techniques of ART.
- *Tumors (fibroids)*: They cause subfertility only when they obstruct lumen of both tubes. This is due to mechanical obstruction of the tubes, but it is not common.

Hostility of Passages to Husband's Spermatozoa

In couples who fail to conceive despite the production of healthy sperms and egg, and there is no obstruction in the passage, there is possibility that the secretions of the vagina are hostile to the husband's sperms.

The hostility may be in the vagina, cervix, or womb.

In such a couple, the husband may have healthy sperms in sufficient number, but the wife fails to conceive because sperms are killed during their passage through the neck of the womb. The secretions may interfere with fertility due to *physical or chemical* changes. The secretions may become too thick and interfere physically with the passage of the sperms.

CAUSES IN FEMALE AND MALE
- Infrequent coitus (sexual intercourse)
- Apareunia
- Painful sexual intercourse

Infrequent Coitus (Sexual Intercourse)
Due to infrequent coitus, the time of production of the egg may be missed in each menstrual cycle. This may be due to a lack of knowledge, or low potency of the husband, social, and professional engagements of the couple.

Erectile Dysfunction
There may be erectile dysfunction (ED) or premature ejaculation (PE).

There could be difficulty in performance of coitus on the part of the male partner. Generally, these difficulties lead to failure of implantation of semen into the vagina. Hence, they need some kind of treatment for these sexual difficulties and for achievement of pregnancy. Physicians can help to overcome these difficulties with psychosexual medical treatment.

Apareunia
The couple may fail to have proper coitus due to sheer ignorance. Sometimes the woman may not relax to allow proper coitus. She may become too tense (vaginismus) and does not allow proper penetration. It may be due to psychological factors, childhood sexual abuse, fear of coitus or due to a local cause.

Painful Sexual Intercourse
In the presence of pelvic infection, endometriosis or any other pelvic disease the coitus may be painful. In such cases semen may not be deposited high up in the front passage of the wife. Sometimes a woman may not relax to allow proper coitus, and complain of pain leading to improper penetration.

CHAPTER 5

Investigations of Subfertility

■ WHEN TO SEEK HELP?

It is generally believed that a healthy young couple living together without use of contraception and practicing coitus 2–3 times a week may take up to 2 years to conceive. In most cases, there is an 80% chance of achieving pregnancy within 1 year.

It is possible that a couple have never conceived (primary subfertility) or they had previously conceived but are finding it difficult to conceive again (secondary subfertility).

If such a couple fails to conceive within 2 years, they should seek help or advice from a doctor or a specialist. In some couples such help is sought earlier. If any of the following conditions is present, instead of waiting for 2 years, the couple may seek advice earlier. They are advised to see a specialist within the 1st year of trying to conceive.

Wife:
- Age >30 years
- Irregular menstruation:
    - Too frequent menstruation, i.e., twice/month
    - Infrequent menstrual cycle, longer than 6 weeks
    - Heavy menstruation
- Previous marriage and subfertility
- History of miscarriages
- History of previous infection in the pelvic organs
- Overweight
- Presence of excessive growth of hair (PCO)
- Presence of any medical disorder
- Using drugs for any medical disorder.

Husband:
- Previous marriage with subfertility
- History of local infection:
    - Urethritis
    - Prostatitis
    - Sexually transmitted infections (STIs)
- Local abnormality:
    - Testes not felt in scrotum
    - Operation for hernia
    - Local swelling

- Coital difficulties [difficulty during sexual intercourse, premature ejaculation (PE), erectile dysfunction (ED)]
- Indulges in excessive smoking or excessive drinking of alcohol
- Using any drugs for medical disease.

■ BEST TIME TO HAVE A BABY

It is strictly personal decision of a couple to decide when to have a baby. If the couple has lived together and tried for a pregnancy for >1 year, then they should have a medical checkup, and if necessary, relevant investigations.

Generally speaking, it is presumed that for a wife the best time to complete her family is between the ages of 20 and 30 years. It is better if she completes her family before the age of 35 years.

Both partners, husband and wife, should be investigated. The investigations of husband are easy to carry out since they carry no risks or side effects. The husband should be investigated first, and the wife should be investigated later.

■ INVESTIGATIONS OF MALE

In order to find out if husband is responsible for the subfertility, the following investigations should be carried out without any omission:
- History
- Physical examination
- Laboratory tests.

History

A complete history is usually taken with special emphasis on the following factors:
- *Age*: Although age is not a very important factor between 20 and 50 years. If the husband is at an advanced age, his fertility gradually starts declining and the desire for sex (libido) and potency may decline.
- *Profession*: If the husband is overworked or psychologically under pressure at work, his libido (desire for sex) will be affected and also his potency and frequency of intercourse. Similarly, if the husband is required to go on tours and travel a lot, he may be missing the time of release of the egg in his wife's cycle.
- *Mumps*: This infection can affect the testes and cause permanent damage leading to their atrophy which causes absence of sperms in the semen (azoospermia).
- Tuberculosis, gonorrhea and other infections can cause a blockage of the narrow tubes that conduct sperms from the testes to urethra, leading to azoospermia.
- History of any injury or operation may cause a blockage of the ducts, or the testes can be damaged due to inflammation or a reduced blood supply **(Fig. 1)**.

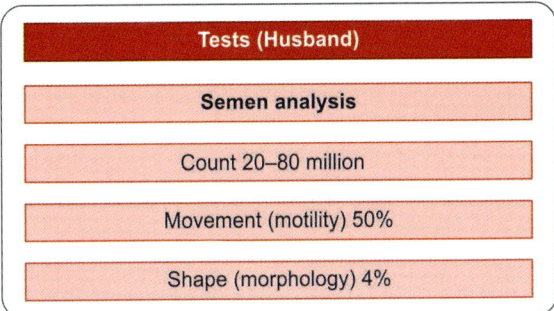

Fig. 1: Husband's test.

- A husband or wife is generally able to explain the problems regarding sexual intercourse. Sometimes they can explain this problem together, but in most cases, it is one partner in isolation, who discloses the correct history.
- If a husband has children from his previous marriage, it does not mean that he is capable of reproduction forever.
- Recent illness, particularly chronic disease, can lead to oligospermia, impotency or lack of libido.
- Intake of drugs due to addiction or for treatment of any disease may affect sperm production or potency in a husband (chemotherapy, drugs for blood pressure, drugs for psychiatric treatment).
- Excessive smoking or drinking of alcohol.

Physical Examination

A thorough general physical examination is carried out. The examination covers all systems, especially the genitalia. The genitalia are examined for any scars, local disease, descent, size, and consistency of testes, presence of dilated blood vessels (varicocele) or fluid (hydrocele), or presence of any discharge from urethra.

Semen Analysis

Before this test is carried out, there should be a gap of coitus (abstinence) for at least 2 days. The specimen may be collected after sexual intercourse or masturbation. Condom is not used to collect the specimen for analysis because condoms usually contain some chemical agent. If a condom is used for collection of specimen, it should be washed thoroughly before use.

The specimen is collected in a clean glass jar and examined after collection. *Initially, the specimen is left on the desk top at room temperature for half an hour.* During this period, the specimen undergoes initial solidification and liquefaction.

The following characteristics of semen are examined:
- Quantity of semen (average 0.2–5 mL)
- *Viscosity*: Normally semen liquefies after half an hour, but if it remains viscous, that could be due to an infection
- Number of sperms per milliliter (average 20–100 million)
- Motility of the spermatozoa (average 50%)
- Shapes of the spermatozoa (>4% are normal in shape)
- Presence of pus cells or any other abnormality
- Absence of fructose or acidic pH of semen suggests blockage within the ejaculatory ducts.

If the test is abnormal, then it should be repeated after a gap of at least a few weeks.

Special Investigations of the Husband

In the case of *absence of spermatozoa in the semen (azoospermia)*, the following special investigations may be carried out:
- *Hormone profile*: The following blood tests are to find out functions of various glands:
  - Thyroid function tests: T_3, T_4, thyroid-stimulating hormone (TSH)
  - Pituitary functions: Follicle-stimulating hormone (FSH), luteinizing hormone (LH), prolactin
  - Testes hormones: Testosterone
  - DNA fragmentation test
  - Sperm survival test.
- *Fine-needle aspiration (FNA) or biopsy of testes*: A needle aspiration biopsy of the testes is carried out under local anesthesia. The aspirate is examined for the presence of spermatozoa. If necessary an open biopsy may be carried out. FNA is a very simple test, practically pain-free, and the husband is not required to stay in the hospital overnight. He goes home after 1–2 hours of the procedure.
- *X-rays of the tubes*: This is a specialized investigation. X-rays are taken after an injection of radio-opaque dye into the male tubes. *This test is used only to identify the site of block in those cases where plastic surgical repair of the block is planned.*
- *Studies of chromosomes (karyotyping)*: This test is only of academic interest. It is carried out to find out the type of chromosomal abnormality. Such abnormalities generally cannot be corrected. This test is advised only for those patients where chromosomal anomaly is suspected.

■ INVESTIGATIONS OF FEMALE

Investigations of the husband should be carried out before the wife's. It should be ensured that there is evidence of sperm production and his capability of fathering a baby.

The following investigations are carried out in all cases of subfertility:
- History
- Physical examination
- Special investigations.

History

A detailed history is obtained, with special emphasis on the following factors:
- *Age*: Fertility is at its peak between the ages of 20 and 25 years. It declines rapidly after the age of 40 years
- Weight and presence of extra hair (hirsutism)
- Duration of marriage and marital relationship; any problems regarding coitus and use of family planning methods (contraception)
- Previous marriages and pregnancies
- Details of menstruation, particularly its regularity or recent change
- Details of previous pregnancies
- Previous infections of genital tract, mumps, operations, and appendicitis or any other infections. Any history of TB, gonorrhea or other STIs
- Any treatment and investigations of subfertility carried out in the past
- Any coital difficulty and frequency per week.

Physical Examination

The examination of the whole body is essential for assessment of general physical health. The following factors are particularly looked into:
- Any recent change in the weight
- Physical feminine features (secondary sexual characters, development of breast, etc.)
- Abnormal distribution of hair or excessive growth of hair
- Abnormal deposition of fat
- Any signs of abnormal function of endocrine glands (thyroid, adrenals)
- All the systems are examined thoroughly for any evidence of local disease
- Local examination will reveal any local abnormality and developmental defect of the genital tract.

Special Investigations of the Wife

Tests of Ovulation (Production of Female Eggs)

The female egg production takes place usually 14 days before the onset of the next menstruation.

After the release of the egg the ovaries produce a special hormone (progesterone). The presence of progesterone in the body confirms the production of egg. The principle of most investigations is to detect production of the egg and find out presence or absence of *progesterone* in the body during second half of menstrual cycle. Usually, this is estimated on 21st day of the cycle by blood test.

The following tests may be carried out to find out the production of the female egg:

- *Basal body temperature (BBT) chart*: If temperature is recorded immediately after waking up in the morning, before getting out of bed, it is called basal body temperature. When this temperature is recorded in a chart, it shows that during first half of the menstrual cycle temperature is at a lower level and during second half of the cycle (after ovulation) temperature is 0.5–1.0°C higher. This test is not used for diagnosis and not recommended now. In the middle of the cycle, ovulation takes place and after a dip for 1 day, the temperature goes up during the subsequent 14 days. This is called biphasic (two phases) temperature chart. It means that if the patient is ovulating, we can reliably work out the day of ovulation. Remember the ovulation date varies from person to person and from one cycle to the next cycle in the same person. Still one gets a reasonably good idea of the date of ovulation, after charting the temperature for 2–3 cycles.
- *Home kit*: This is an "ovulation predictor kit". The principle of this test is to detect the release of a LH called "surge of LH hormone". When there is a sudden increase of LH levels in the body, ovulation or release of egg takes place within 12–24 hours.

    The test strip is usually used twice a day, in the morning and evening. The strip detects LH in the urine. When the kit gives a positive result for LH surge, it means ovulation will take place within 12–24 hours. Accordingly, sexual intercourse can be planned.
- *Self-test of cervical mucus*: The neck of the womb (cervix) produces thick secretions which keep the passage blocked. The thickness of these secretions changes during different days of the menstrual cycle.

    Soon after menstruation ends, these secretions are thick but just a day before ovulation (release of egg) these secretions become watery like the white of an egg.

    A woman can check these secretions by placing her finger in the front passage every day, and record the thickness in a chart. Watery secretion means ovulation day is close. A woman can work out the day of ovulation in her menstrual cycle by checking the consistency of these secretions.

The above mentioned tests are simple and can be easily carried out by the patient at home. Doctors conduct much more elaborate tests to find out ovulation.

These tests are: **(Fig. 2)**
- Ultrasound, especially transvaginal sonography (TVS)
- Hormonal estimation of estradiol and progesterone levels

Ultrasonography (TVS)

This is the most convenient procedure that helps track the growth of a female egg in the ovary, and it also helps to find out, when the ovum is ripe to be shed by the ovary.

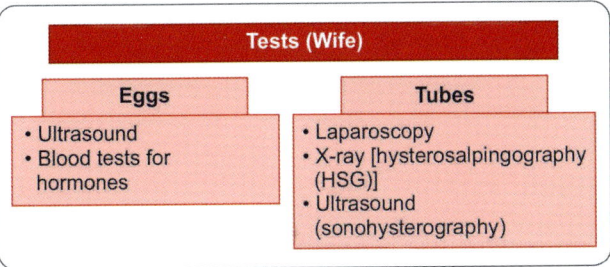

Fig. 2: Tests for female.

This is more reliable than most of the other tests for this purpose, especially when carried out through vagina. This method of ultrasonography is called TVS.

Generally, this method is used in those cases where close monitoring of ovarian stimulation and follicular growth is required [in vitro fertilization (IVF) or test tube baby treatment].

Hormone Profile

The tests described for evaluation of hormones in the male are also carried out in female. In addition to those tests, estrogens, progesterone, and fasting insulin are also evaluated.

Progesterone test
This hormone is produced in the human body only if ovulation takes place. If a small amount of blood is drawn on the 21st day of the menstrual cycle, and tested in a laboratory, it can confirm the presence of progesterone in the blood, ovulation can be confirmed.

Pipelle test
This is an outpatient procedure carried out by a special narrow plastic cannula (catheter). This special cannula helps to collect a few pieces of the lining of the cavity of the womb, with the help of vacuum created by a syringe. If the test is carried out just before the onset of menstruation, shows certain changes, which confirm the diagnosis of ovulation (secretory changes). This is a painless procedure, performed without anesthesia, in the outpatient clinic.

Biopsy of lining of the womb (Endometrial Biopsy or D & C)
Changes in the lining provide very useful information regarding production of the egg.

This test is carried out in an operating room under general anesthesia. In this test, a small piece of the lining of the womb is taken out, after dilating the neck of the womb. This piece is sent to a laboratory for examination under a microscope (histopathology). *This test was previously carried out for detection of production of the egg but with availability of other simple tests, it is not necessary any more.* The drawback of this test is that the patient has to be admitted into a hospital for at least 1 day, and she has to go through general anesthesia.

Investigations of Subfertility

Laparoscopy
The presence of corpus luteum (changes in the ovary after ovulation) provides visual evidence of ovulation. Similarly, a corpus luteum may be seen at laparotomy.

Most Common Tests

To find out whether ovulation is taking place or not, ultrasonography, especially TVS and *21st day progesterone* test are most commonly used in the workup of subfertility.

Tests for Patency of the Tubes

The obstruction or blockage of both tubes is one of the most common causes of subfertility in Asian countries. The following are tubal patency tests carried out for investigations of subfertility.

Tubal Insufflation Test (D and I)

This test is obsolete and not used these days. We have described this test because some gynecologists still use it. This test is called Rubin's test after the name of Rubin who described this test in 1920.

In this test, air or carbon dioxide gas is injected into the uterine cavity under pressure. If tubes are patent, gas escapes into abdominal cavity through the openings of the tubes and pressure in the uterine cavity falls. On the other hand, if both tubes are blocked, there is no leakage of the gas and its pressure, seen in the manometer, is maintained.

This test is preferably carried out during the first half of the menstrual cycle, i.e., a few days after cessation of the menstrual flow.

Usually, no anesthesia is required for this test, but it should be carried out under aseptic conditions (operating theater). *This test carries the risk of embolism and is not very reliable.*

Sonohysterography

In this test, normal saline is injected into the uterine cavity through the neck of the womb which is approached through vagina.

The flow of fluid is visualized by ultrasonography, preferably by TVS. The escape of fluid through the tubes into the abdominal cavity can be easily seen and documented by a photograph. If the tubes are blocked, then there is no flow of fluid into the tubes and abdominal cavity.

X-rays [Hysterosalpingography (HSG)] (Figs. 3 to 5)

This is another test for patency of the fallopian tubes. In this test, a radio-opaque dye is injected into the uterine cavity and X-rays are taken to see the shadow of the cavity and the fallopian tubes. The test causes some degree

Investigations of Subfertility

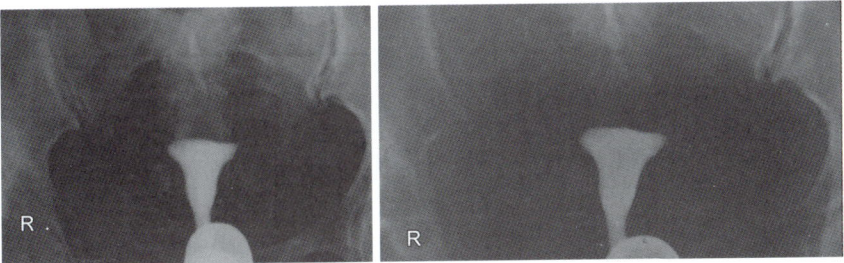

Fig. 3: Cornual block.

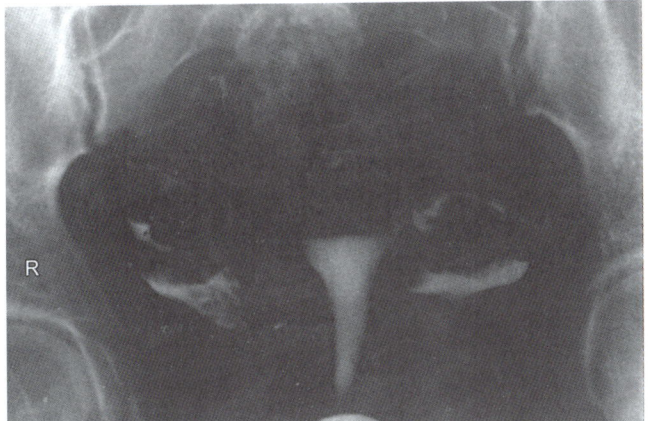

Fig. 4: Patent tubes.

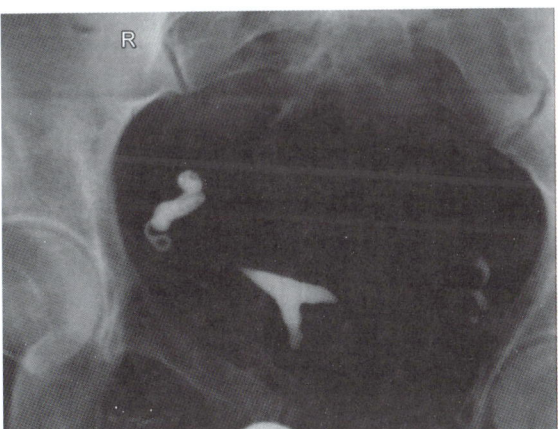

Fig. 5: Fimbrial block with hydrosalpinx.

of discomfort or pain. The procedure is basically the same as used for sonohysterography test. In this test, a solution of radiopaque dye is injected and X-rays are taken.

Investigations of Subfertility

Laparoscopy

This procedure is carried out in an operating theater under general anesthesia. A small incision near the umbilicus is made. During laparoscopy, methylene blue or any other dye may be injected through the uterine cannula and free spill of the dye in abdominal cavity is visualized. In patients with blocked fallopian tubes, there is no spill of dye.

Laparoscopy gives an opportunity to see the inside of the abdominal cavity. It provides opportunity to see the pelvic organs (uterus, ovaries, and fallopian tubes) and assess their health. There may be a minor or early disease which cannot be felt on physical examination or detected by ultrasonography, i.e., adhesions, endometriosis, and small myomas (fibroids), etc. In the workup of subfertility, laparoscopy gives the most comprehensive opportunity of evaluating the pelvic organs. Remember that this is an invasive test, and should be carried out in operating theater, under general anesthesia, by an expert surgeon.

During any laparotomy, to test the patency of the tubes, an injection of methylene blue, as in laparoscopy, can also be carried out.

PLAN OF ORGANIZED INVESTIGATIONS (FLOWCHARTS 1 AND 2)

The following plan will help to complete almost all the relevant tests of the subfertile couple in the shortest period. 1st day of menstruation is called day one:

Day 1: Husband's semen analysis provided, there is a gap in coitus abstinence of at least 2 days.

Flowchart 1: Algorithm for basic evaluation.

Basic evaluation at first visit
- History
  - Menstrual history
  - Sexual history
  - Past medical/surgical history
  - Past infertility treatment history
  - Family history
- Examination
  - Breast, height, weight, BMI, waist circumference
  - For acne and hirsutism
  - Per abdominal and PS and PV
  - Transvaginal ultrasound
    - *Cervix*: Length and curvature
    - *Uterus*: Length, width, and AP
    - *Pathology*: Polyp, fibroids, adenomyosis, Mullerian anomalies, endometrial thickness, and pattern correlated with the day of MC
    - *Ovaries*: Measurement and volume, AFC (2–9 mm) on Day 2/3, presence or absence of cyst
    - Mobility of uterus and ovaries (sliding slide)
    - *POD*: Tethered/obliterated/collection

(AFC: antral follicle count; AP: anteroposterior; BMI: body mass index; MC: menstrual cycle)

Investigations of Subfertility

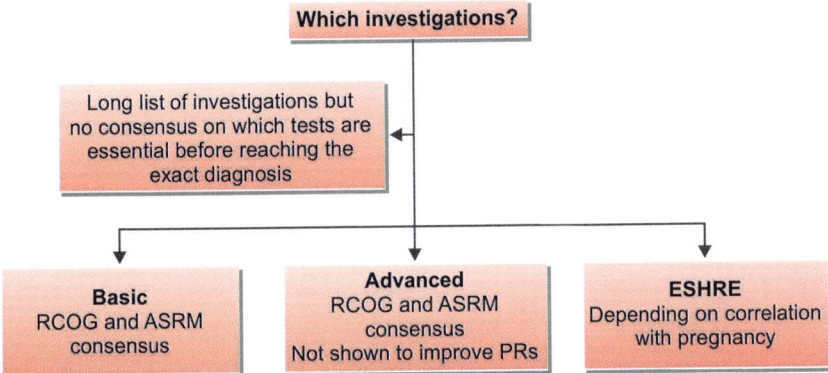

Flowchart 2: RCOG/ASRM/ESHRE guideline.

(RCOG: Royal College of Obstetrics and Gynaecology; ASRM: American Society of Reproductive Medicine; ESHRE: European Society of Human Reproduction and Embryology)

Day 2: If necessary, wife's hormone estimation (FSH, LH, PRL, estradiol, etc.).
Day 14–16: Postcoital test (PCT) (rarely required)
Day 21: Blood test for progesterone levels
Next cycle (if necessary):
Day 5–10: Sonohysterography or hysterosalpingography or laparoscopy.

CHAPTER 6
Treatment of Subfertility (Female Factors)

■ INTRODUCTION

With recent advances in investigations, and treatment of subfertility, a lot of progress has been made. Those patients who were previously declared subfertile can now be helped, and successfully treated.

■ FEMALE FACTORS (FIG. 1)

The treatment of the wife depends upon the causative factor. The line of treatment is as follows:
- Explanation and reassurance (counseling)
- Improvement of general health
- Treatment of infrequent or absent ovulation (induction of ovulation)
- Treatment of hostility of vagina
- Treatment of blocked tubes
    - Surgery
    - In vitro fertilization (IVF)/intracytoplasmic sperm injection(ICSI)/ embryo transfer (ET)

Counseling (Explanation and Reassurance) (Flowchart 1)

Subfertile women are under a lot of social pressure, from family members, society and even friends. They tend to be psychologically stressed and emotionally upset. *They need emotional support.*

The most important reassurance is to provide them with the information that they can be helped medically. Even in those cases where the exact cause of subfertility cannot be determined (*unexplained subfertility*) simple drugs like

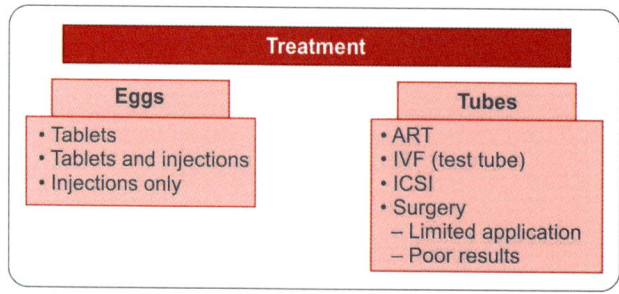

Fig. 1: Treatment plan.
(ART: assisted reproductive technique; ICSI: intracytoplasmic sperm injection; IVF: in vitro fertilization)

Treatment of Subfertility (Female Factors)

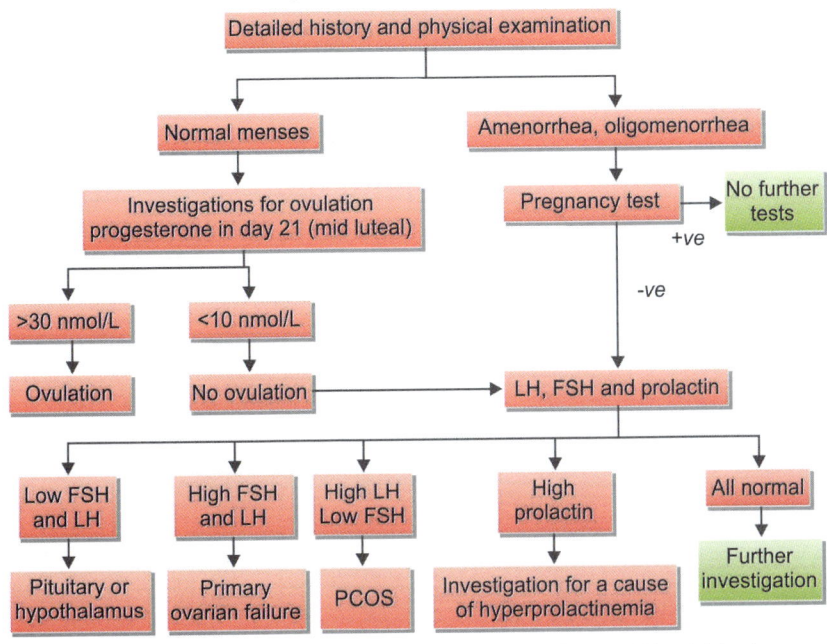

Flowchart 1: Diagnostic approach to subfertility in females.

(FSH: follicle-stimulating hormone; PCOS: polycystic ovarian syndrome; LH: luteinizing hormone)

clomiphene citrate (CC) or if need be IVF or ICSI can offer a solution. These methods are not only therapeutic (treatment) but in some cases, diagnostic (tests to find out the cause of *subfertility*). In case of failure of treatment, the couple needs counseling about life without children.

While undergoing treatment, the couple should be counseled about *how to overcome stress*. There should be special counseling sessions, regarding the management of stress. *They need emotional, psychological, social, and financial support.*

Improvement in General Health

In Pakistan, particularly in the lower income group, the health of women is generally poor. It can be improved by the following measures:
- Correction of dietary habits
- Advice regarding hygiene
- Correction of anemia
- Treatment of any chronic infection or disease
- Reduction in weight (if necessary).

Induction of Ovulation (Controlled Stimulation of Ovaries)

Before embarking upon this mode of treatment, it must be ensured, through all available means **(Flowchart 2)**, that the cause of subfertility is only *failure of production of the female egg or unexplained subfertility*. This treatment is expensive

Treatment of Subfertility (Female Factors)

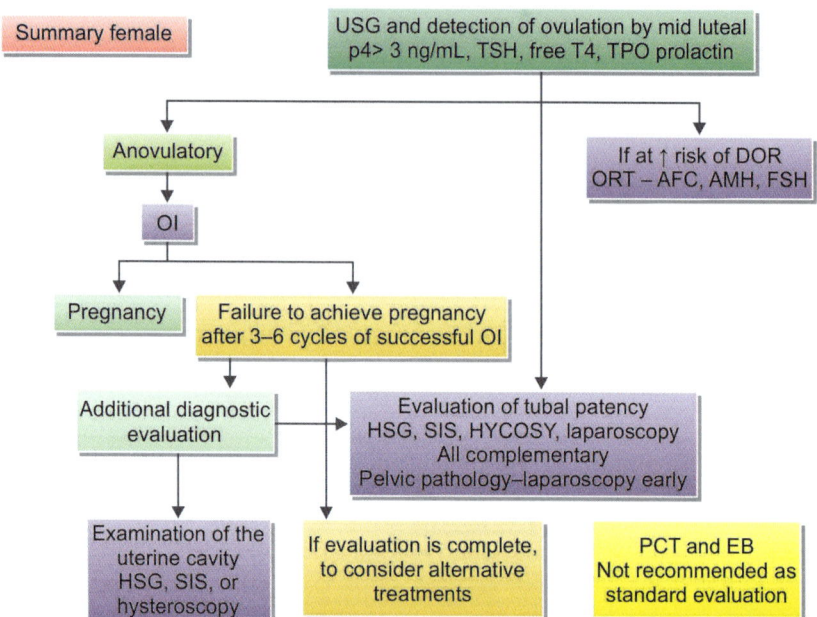

Flowchart 2: Evaluation of absent ovulation.

(AFC: antral follicle count; AMH: anti-mullerian hormone; FSH: follicle-stimulating hormone; HSG: hysterosalpingography; PCT: postcoital test; SIS: saline infused sonography; TPO: thyroid peroxidase; TSH: thyroid-stimulating hormone)

and carries certain risks for the patient. The ovaries can be stimulated by the following methods **(Flowchart 3)**:

- Metformin
- Clomiphene citrate
- Aromatase inhibitors
- Injections
- Gonadotropins
- Laparoscopic ovarian diathermy (LOD).

Metformin

Those patients who have PCO/PCOS (polycystic ovarian syndrome), and have high fasting insulin levels can be initially treated by a course of metformin tablets continuously for 3–6 months. Some of them respond to this simple treatment by menstruating regularly, ovulating and becoming pregnant.

Aromatase Inhibitors

- Letrozole is a fertility drug to stimulate and/or regulate ovulation.
- Letrozole is an aromatase inhibitor and works by lowering the production of estrogen.

Flowchart 3: Treatment of infrequent absent ovulation.

GnRH
- Indicated only in hypothalamic hypogonadism
- GnRh therapy with use of micropumps
- SC/IV administration with micropumps for several months makes compliance difficult

Gonadotropin therapy
- Indicated only in hypothalamic hypogonadism with low FSH and LH levels
- Dose: hCG - 2000 IU twice a weekb FSH – 75 IU thrice a week
- Given for 3 months
- First spermatozoa appear in the ejaculate after a median of 7 months

Anti-estrogen therapy- CC/Tamoxifen
- Block the estrogen receptor preventing inhibition of GT secretion
- Most controversial results—some studies report benefit, while others do not
- CC – 25 mg or Tamoxifen 20 mg for 6 months. Tamoxifen is preferred to CC as it exerts a weaker estrogenic action
- Establishment of clear cut guidelines for use necessary

(CC: clomiphene citrate; FSH: follicle-stimulating hormone; GnRH: gonadotropin-releasing hormone; hCG: human chorionic gonadotropin; IV: intravenous; LH: luteinizing hormone; SC: subcutaneous)

- *Dose*: Take letrozole from day 2 to day 6 and organize an USS between day 10 and 14 of the cycle.
- Generally has mild side effects, e.g.,
  - Mood swings
  - Nausea, vomiting
  - Headache
  - Blurring of vision
  - Fatigue
  - Muscle aches.

Clomiphene Citrate

This is a nonsteroidal compound. *Clomiphene is a drug of choice*, for stimulation of ovaries in cases, where some ovarian activity is present, with normal or subnormal production of hormones by the pituitary gland. It is a safer drug as compared to gonadotropins. The incidence of hyperstimulation and OHSS is low after treatment with clomiphene.

Clomiphene has been most successfully used in the treatment of subfertility due to absence of production of female eggs in the ovaries. In addition to this, it has produced good results in unexplained subfertility, amenorrhea following administration of contraceptive pills.

Administration:
After thorough investigations and *confirmation of the fact that there is a failure of production of female eggs*, the following regimen is followed:

One or two tablet of CC 50–100 mg is given for 5 days. Ovulation occurs 5–7 days after the last day of intake of the drug.

If there is no response to the treatment and ovulation fails to occur, then the following month in the next cycle CC is repeated for 5 days at increased dosage (100–150 mg daily).

The treatment is monitored, usually, by vaginal ultrasound (TVS), carried out between 9 and 13 days. This serial sonographic follow-up is called (follicle tracking). When the follicles seem to be ripe, then in some patients, Inj of hCG 5,000 or 10,000 units may be given to force shedding of the ova. *This injection is not necessary for all patients.*

The monitoring may also be carried out by maintaining a temperature chart (BBT) or by a cycle day 21 progesterone test. The response is good, if more than one follicle is stimulated and multiple eggs are produced.

After induction of ovulation, due to the formation of multiple follicles, the risk of multiple pregnancy (twins, triplets) is more common (nearly 10%).

If there is no response, then the course is repeated with 4 tablets (200 mg) daily, during the next month. If there is no response after the third course, then the treatment is usually discontinued.

During administration of clomiphene (CC) the patient is told of the possible day of ovulation and advised to have sexual intercourse during the period of 5th to 7th day after the last day of the tablets.

Before initiating the next course the patient is examined for any ovarian enlargement. If there is any palpable or sonographic ovarian enlargement, the treatment may be discontinued or postponed for 1–2 months.

Side effects:
The following side effects are seen:
- *Heat flash*: This is a common side effect, 5–10% of patients complain of heat flash at the end of the course (like menopausal syndrome). This does not happen in each cycle of the treatment.
- *Hyperstimulation of the ovaries*: It is uncommon with this treatment.
- *Multiple pregnancies*: Ten percent of patients treated with clomiphene conceive twin pregnancies.

Gonadotropins

The gonadotropins may be used for stimulation of the ovaries. Their use is restricted to those cases where other alternative treatments have failed. They are used in centers where facilities for close follow-up by ultrasound (TVS) or hormone estimation are available. In most of the assisted reproductive technique (ART) patients injections of gonadotropins are used.

Contraindications:
Generally, they are the same as for clomiphene except that gonadotropins can be given to the patients with the pituitary failure whereas CC cannot be prescribed to these patients.

Side effects:
The side effects in cases of gonadotropin therapy are more frequent and more severe as compared to clomiphene stimulation.
- *Overstimulation of the ovaries [ovarian hyperstimulation syndrome (OHSS)]:* Even with careful monitoring, the incidence of severe hyperstimulation (OHSS) is still 3–4%. This could be minimized with close monitoring. The ovaries are over stimulated and multiple large cysts are formed. The cysts may rupture or hemorrhage, with serious consequences, requiring surgery.

    The sudden enlargement of the cysts may cause formation of ascites, or hydrothorax, and cause dehydration resulting in changes in the chemistry of the blood. *This requires hospitalization and intensive medical treatment.*
- *Multiple births (twins, triplets):* The incidence of multiple births is >10%. With careful selection of dosage the incidence is reduced.

Gonadotropin preparations and administration:
Gonadotropins are given by injections. They are procured by three methods:
1. Urine of postmenopausal women
2. Urine of pregnant women
3. Prepared artificially in the laboratory (recombinant)

There are three types of preparations available in the market:
1. *Urinary human menopausal gonadotropins (HMGs)*: They contain two hormones FSH and LH, almost equal doses of both. Each ampoule contains 75 IU of FSH and LH.
2. *Purified HMG*: This is procured from urine of pregnant women but contents are purified to achieve better results. Each ampoule contains FSH 75 units but still some impurity of LH is present.
3. *Laboratory synthetic preparation (recombinant)*: This is a pure preparation of FSH without any other contamination. This is the most effective and reliable but the *most expensive preparation.*

Other Drugs Used during Stimulation of Ovaries

The following drugs are also used during induction of ovulation:
- GnRH analogs
- GnRH antagonists

When GnRH analogs/antagonists are used these drugs suppress production of gonadotropins from the pituitary gland. This helps to control ovarian stimulation by the external injections of gonadotropins. Due to better control, the stimulation of ovaries is better regulated.

Protocol of Stimulation

During subfertility treatment, the following regimens are used for induction of ovulation, [controlled ovarian stimulation (COS)].
- Clomiphene citrate only
- Clomiphene citrate and Inj hCG (CC + Inj hCG)
- CC + Inj HMG + Inj hCG
- Long or short protocol:
  - Inj GnRH (analog) + Inj HMG + Inj hCG
  - Inj GnRH (analog) + Inj purified HMG + Inj hCG
  - Inj GnRH (analog) + Inj recombinant FSH+ Inj hCG or Inj LH® (long protocol start on CD21)
  - Inj GnRH (antagonist) + Inj recombinant FSH + Inj hCG or Inj LH® (short protocol start on CD2)

In case of long protocol, the treatment starts on the 21st day of the menstrual cycle and generally lasts for 2–3 weeks.

In case of short protocol, the treatment starts on the 2nd day of the menstrual cycle and it lasts for 10–14 days. This is called COS. It is used for intrauterine insemination (IUI), IVF, or ICSI treatments.

This stimulation helps to produce a large number of eggs. In case of IVF/ICSI they are picked up for IVF and subsequently either fertilized eggs are put back into the uterine cavity ET or frozen embryo transfer (FET) (cryopreserved) for use in the later months.

Laparoscopic Ovarian Diathermy

If the wife has polycystic ovarian disease or syndrome (*PCO or PCOS*) then she most probably has infrequent ovulation or absence of ovulation. Such a situation is helped by giving metformin, CC tablets or gonadotropins. If repeated attempts to stimulate the ovaries fail to produce adequate stimulation then multiple small follicles can be diathermized with the help of a laparoscope. Monopolar diathermy should be used minimally. It has negative effect on ovaries in later age.

Generally, the response is immediate and spontaneous ovulation may take place. This response is not permanents, attempts to help the wife to become pregnant after LOD should follow immediately.

■ TREATMENT OF CLOSED/BLOCKED TUBES IN FEMALES

The patients with closed blocked fallopian tubes can be helped by one of the following two methods:
- Surgery (laparoscopic or conventional)
- ARTs [assisted reproductive techniques (IVF, ICSI)]

Before embarking upon surgical treatment to open female tubes, it must be ensured that there is no other causative factor for subfertility. The husband is investigated, and it is made certain that he is healthy and his semen analysis is normal. Similarly, it is ensured that the wife's ovaries are functioning and rest of the genital tract is healthy. It is ascertained that there is no other defect contributing toward subfertility.

- After eliminating all other factors, the site and type of blockage is identified by X-rays (hysterosalpingography). Surgical correction of the tubes may be carried out by laparotomy or by laparoscopy.
- The results are better if the block is due to previous sterilization operation [bilateral tubal ligation (BTL)]. On the other hand, the results are poor if both tubes are blocked due to tuberculosis or other infections.

The results of microsurgical treatment of blockage of the female tubes are 30–70% if performed by a competent surgeon.

Assisted Reproductive Techniques

See Chapter 7

Treatment of Other Causes of Subfertility

The following factors, which may only be partially responsible for causing subfertility, are treated accordingly.

- *Congenital defects of the genital tract*: All the congenital defects, especially if they cause difficulties during intercourse, are dealt with surgically. Rigid hymen and vaginal septum can be excised. Narrow introitus can be enlarged by operation or stretching under general anesthesia.
- *Infections*: Vaginitis, cervicitis, and inflammations of any other part of the genital tract are eradicated as soon as possible. Infection of the front passage, the neck of the womb are treated with antibiotics and other local drugs.
- *Prolapse*: In a few cases, laxity of the walls of the front passage (prolapse) is responsible for subfertility. *If all other factors are eliminated, then correction of this condition may improve chances of fertility.*
- *Tumors*: If there is a tumor (fibroid), it may be removed by an operation. *In most of the patients this operation is not required.*
- *Cervical mucus hostility*: Where the causative factor is only cervical secretion (mucus) hostility, the following advice may be given.

  The husband is advised to use a condom during coitus for 6 months or so. It is hoped that by avoiding contact of sperms with the secretory glands of the neck of the womb, the titer of antibodies may fall. On resumption of coitus without condom the sperms may be able to pass through the neck of the womb without being attacked by the antibodies. In case of failure of this treatment IUI is advised.
- *Weight*: The best results of subfertility treatment are obtained if a woman is of an average weight, body mass index (BMI) 18–29. In case she is underweight, after exclusion of medical causes for being under weight, she should be advised about correct diet and exercises.

The most common feature in subfertile women is being *overweight*. In the majority of women, it is due to PCO but in others it could be depression, leading to over eating and gain in weight. After exclusion of medical causes of being overweight, the patient needs advice from a dietician who can help her to reduce weight. Generally, weight reduction is difficult, particularly in PCOS, but with the help of a dietician and willing cooperation of the patient, it is possible to bring the BMI within normal range or lose at least 5% of her original weight.

Intrauterine Insemination

The IUI involves implantation of sperms directly into the uterine cavity with a syringe and narrow uterine cannula so that the secretions of the neck of the womb are bypassed. Those patients who have patent fallopian tubes, and reasonably satisfactory semen analysis, can be helped by this simple procedure. The success rate is generally quoted as 5–15%. It is cost effective, and causes least inconvenience. In most of the centers, it costs only 25,000–35,000 rupees. The induction of ovulation is carried out by CC or Inj HMG which keeps the drug cost very low. The procedure requires 2–3 visits, for TVS monitoring of stimulation, and IUI.

The semen can be obtained from two sources:
1. Donor
2. Husband

In case of nonobstructive azoospermia, (absence of husband's sperm production in testes) some body else's sperms (donor) can be injected, *but it is not practiced in Pakistan*. Husband must be willing for this type of insemination because legally this is illegitimate pregnancy.

IUI with donor semen has religious, social, moral, and legal complications. The author has never used donor sperms for IUI or IVF/ICSI.

The use of donor sperms is practiced in most of the western countries as well as India and Nepal.

Indications for Intrauterine Insemination

- Severe hostility due to secretions of the neck of the womb which cannot be overcome by abstinence or use of condom.
- Gross deformity of husband which makes it impossible for him to plant semen into front passage [impotency, sexual difficulty (SD) or erectile difficulty (ED), or premature ejaculation (PE), hypospadias, etc.].
- Oligospermia (moderately low sperm count)
- *Unexplained subfertility.*

Procedure

Intrauterine insemination is carried out as follows:
- Selection of patients
- Ovarian stimulation (COS)

- Monitoring (TVS)
- Intrauterine sperm injection
- Follow-up.

Selection of patients:
Selection of patients for IUI is made carefully. It is ensured by detailed investigations that there is an indication for IUI. It is also ascertained that all conditions for IUI are fulfilled. Generally, IUI is carried out for the couples where semen analysis shows sperm count of >10 million/mL with reasonable motility. If count is lower than sperm survival test is carried out to find out the number of surviving sperms after 24 hours of incubation (*see* Chapter 7). If the surviving sperms are >3 million, only then IUI may be recommended. In case the count is lower than IVF/ICSI are preferred.

The other important requirement is patency of the fallopian tubes. It should be ensured that the tubes are patent or at least one tube is healthy.

The treatment modalities should be explained to the couple. Although overall cost of IUI is not very high yet the failure or success rates should be discussed. In most of the centers IUI success rate is 5–15%. The success rate seems to be low but as compared to the cost of IVF/ICSI it is cost-effective.

It goes without saying that the wife should be healthy to carry pregnancy without any serious medical problems. It should be hammered again and again *that sperms used for IUI procedure shall belong to the husband only*. No donor sperms are used under any circumstances. This is particularly important because some couples/husbands may have a wrong notion or misgiving that somebody else's sperms may be used, especially in a case of severe oligospermia or azoospermia.

The couple is advised to abstain from coitus after 10th day of the cycle.

Ovarian stimulation:
Controlled ovarian stimulation may be carried out by any of the methods described on Chapter 7. Usually for IUI one of the following regimens is used:
- CC only
- CC + Inj hCG
- CC + Inj HMG + Inj hCG

Generally, *long and short protocols* are not used, however, there is no contraindication for their use. These stimulation regimens could be used in those patients who fail to respond to the above mentioned regimens.

Monitoring:
The patients for IUI need careful monitoring but in view of the stimulation regimens used for these patients it need not be as close as for short and long protocols. Generally, ultrasound (TVS) monitoring is adequate in these patients. The objectives of monitoring are to find out the following:
- Optimum stimulation
- Time for sperm injection

In most of the centers, TVS monitoring is carried out as follows:
- First TVS assessment of the ovaries is carried out prior to stimulation. This will ensure the status of ovaries without stimulation and also rule out presence of any abnormality, i.e., PCO or cyst.
- Second TVS is mostly performed between 10 and 12 days of the cycle. It shows the degree of stimulation and size of the leading follicle. If the size of follicles is smaller than the recommended size then another TVS is needed.
- Third TVS is carried out 1–2 days after the second assessment. If TVS shows adequate stimulation then the patient is advised to return for sperm injection or Inj hCG is given which is followed by sperm injection within 24–36 hours.
- Fourth TVS is *occasionally required*, especially in those cases where Inj hCG is not given. This is usually 1–2 days after the sperm injection. This TVS will show disappearance of the leading follicle which confirms ovulation.

Intrauterine sperm injection:
After second or third TVS patient is advised about the date and time for IUI. The couple is advised to arrive in the morning. The husband gives the specimen of his semen. He is advised to observe care as described in Chapter 7. The semen is processed in the IVF laboratory. Only 0.1–0.2 mL of the prepared specimen is loaded in a special syringe and it is injected into the uterine cavity through the neck of the womb using a special cannula. This is a painless procedure and it does not require any anesthesia. After the injection the patient may rest for 15–30 minutes. Later she can walk and go home; she does not need any special care or medicines.

■ FOLLOW-UP

After the intrauterine injection the patient can continue her normal life. There is no need for any special care. She needs to send her urine for pregnancy test after 14 days of IUI. The chances of positive report are only 5–15%.

In view of minimal inconvenience and very low cost, failure does not upset the patients as much as after IVF/ICSI.

If the test is positive the patient needs no special care. She needs same care as after a spontaneous pregnancy. In case of failure, the procedure can be repeated after a gap of 1–2 months. Psychological support during this period helps the patient to overcome depression sooner.

This procedure may be repeated 3–4 times. After repeated failure the couple may be advised to go on for IVF/ICSI. The accumulated success after 3–4 attempts is higher, may be up to 20–25%.

CHAPTER 7

Assisted Reproductive Techniques (Test Tube Baby)

■ INTRODUCTION

In medical terminology, this is also known as in vitro fertilization (IVF), i.e., fertilization outside the human body.

It means that the pregnancy or fertilization of female egg takes places outside the human body. Within 2-5 days after fertilization, the fertilized egg (embryo) is transferred into the womb of the patient and the baby grows inside the womb of its mother. The fertilized egg (embryo) spends only first 2-5 days outside the human body and rest of the period is spent inside the womb, in the same manner as after a spontaneous natural pregnancy.

In certain cases where the factors responsible for subfertility of a couple are blockage of the tubes in the wife, the union of sperm and female egg cannot take place. In such cases, female eggs are collected from the ovary through a special technique, and they are kept in a dish in an incubator. The husband's semen is collected and is processed. Later the sperms, about 100,000-150,000, from the processed specimen of husband are added to the dish containing wife's eggs. After 2-5 days, the fertilized eggs (embryos) are put back into the cavity of the womb. Usually, 1-2 embryos are put back into the womb. These days, in most of the centers, even a single embryo is used (SET). The union of the husband's sperms and wife's egg takes place in the incubator. After 24 hours, the eggs are inspected under a microscope for evidence of fertilization. Later, after 1-4 days, they are put into the womb, embryos continue to grow inside the uterine cavity for the rest of the gestation period. If implantation does not take place then the embryos die (degenerate).

There are many centers in the world where subfertile couples are being helped by this technique. But unfortunately even in the best centers the success rate is only 50-70%. This low success rate could be due to some deficiency in the techniques, or it is a natural protection against abnormal eggs and spermatozoa.

After the embryo transfer (ET), the patients are provided support, with vaginal progesterone tablets for the initial 16-20 weeks of pregnancy. The patient has to use these tablets through the front passage (vagina) every day. In case the pregnancy test is negative then after the 14th day of ET, vaginal bleeding takes place, this means the treatment has failed or pregnancy has not been achieved. In such a situation the vaginal tablets of progesterone should be discontinued.

Till now more than million babies have been delivered in the world with assisted reproductive technique (ART). The incidence of *malformation* among these babies is nearly the same as in rest of the population. There should be no anxiety on this account. However, the risks of multiple pregnancies and early pregnancy loss are higher than in the general population. As regards multiple pregnancy it is recommended that, if possible, only one embryo should be used at the time of embryo transfer (SET).

In our country, even this success rate is a great help. Due to extensive damage to the tubes by infection most of the patients with blocked tubes cannot be helped by surgery. This is where ART can help the subfertile couples.

INDICATIONS

- Blocked tubes
- Absent or infrequent ovulation
- Husband's low count (oligospermia) or obstructive azoospermia
- Unexplained subfertility
- Endometriosis
- Repeated failure of intrauterine insemination (IUI).

Steps of Assisted Reproductive Technique

- Selection and counseling of the patient
- Controlled ovarian stimulation
- Monitoring of ovaries
- Ovum pick up (OPU, retrieval of eggs)
- Semen preparation and insemination
- Laboratory procedures
- Embryo transfer
- Luteal phase support.

Stages of Assisted Reproductive Technique

1. Controlled stimulation of ovaries (COS)
2. Retrieval of eggs or OPU
3. Insemination/fertilization
4. Embryo transfer
5. Implantation.

SELECTION AND COUNSELING OF PATIENT FOR ASSISTED REPRODUCTIVE TECHNIQUE

Assisted reproductive technique is an extremely *stressful treatment*. It may prove to be emotionally as well as financially taxing. Generally, the cost, including drugs and disposables, ranges between rupees two hundred thousand to three hundred and fifty thousand rupees (200,000–350,000). The expense varies mostly due to the cost of drugs used for ovarian stimulation and other expenses add up to cost 500,000 or more.

The success rate of achieving a pregnancy is also not very high. It ranges between 60 and 70%. Take home baby rate is even lower because of a high rate of early pregnancy loss (miscarriage, ectopic pregnancy, and complications). Once pregnancy is established the incidence of complications is the same as after a spontaneous natural pregnancy.

Keeping in view the high cost, and low success rates, a careful evaluation of patients age, financial status and psychological make up should be carried out. In case of failure a patient may experience depression. The financial loss due to unsuccessful treatment can contribute to depression.

Before embarking on this treatment all of the medical problems of the wife should be excluded and treated. The couple should be counseled to accept failure as a possible outcome of the treatment. Before starting of the treatment hormonal assessment of the wife and local evaluation of her genital tract are necessary. It goes without saying that appropriate psychological assessment should be made. In case of failure such help should be available.

The treatment modalities should be explained to the couple. Various choices should be discussed, so that the couple has an opportunity of making a choice. If there is any other available choice, it should be explained and offered to them. The couple should be helped to make an appropriate choice according to their financial status and emotional needs. Once the treatment is started, they should be advised to relax and pray for the best.

■ OVARIAN STIMULATION

To procure more ova for higher chances of success almost all patients for ART need COS. Although the first IVF baby of the world, Louise Browne, was born without ovarian stimulation by natural cycle. Today the natural cycle ART is practiced at very few centers.

Various stimulation regimens, used all over the world, are described in Chapter 6.

In Pakistan, usually one of the following regimens is recommended:
- CC + Inj HMG + Inj hCG
- Long Protocol start on CD21
  - Inj GnRH (a) + Inj HMG + Inj hCG
  - Inj GnRH (a) + Inj Recombinant FSH + Inj hCG

Protocol

See Antagonist protocol (Chapter 6).

MONITORING OF STIMULATION

During ovarian stimulation a patient requires very close supervision and monitoring. The objectives are twofold:
- To achieve optimum number of mature eggs
- To detect and treat any serious complications of ovarian stimulation.

The monitoring is usually by either ultrasonography through the front passage [transvaginal sonography (TVS)] which is usually carried out on 4th, 6th, 10th, 11th, and 12th days of injections of gonadotropins (Inj HMG or Inj FSH®). The frequency of TVS can be adjusted according to patient's response.

During ultrasound monitoring, the number of follicles in both ovaries and their growth rates are evaluated. When size of the leading follicle reaches 18–20 mm, it is considered to be the right time to give 5,000 units or 10,000 units hCG injection. After this injection, all injections of FSH and GnRH are stopped.

OVUM PICK-UP

After the hCG injection, within 34–36 hours, the patient is taken to the operating theater. All available eggs are sucked out of the ovaries under ultrasonographic (TVS) guidance with the help of a special long and narrow needle. Generally, this procedure is carried out under local anesthesia and it takes about 30–45 minutes, the patient may feel slight discomfort at the time of the needle punctures of the vagina or ovarian follicles.

In case of good stimulation, 6–10 eggs are procured. The patient can go home after a couple of hours.

SEMEN PREPARATION

Immediately after the eggs are picked up from the wife's ovaries, the husband is requested to provide a specimen of his semen in a sterile container. He is advised to wash himself with water only, and not to use soap or any other lubricant for masturbation. He should be advised to ensure that ejaculate is collected carefully in the jar and not to spill it during collection. It is recommended that before giving the specimen he should abstain from coitus for 2 days.

The specimen is left on the desk top, at room temperature, for half an hour. During this period, initially, the semen consolidates and later liquefies. After liquefaction the usual semen parameters are examined. Then it is added to the semen preparation medium and centrifuged to make a pellet of the spermatozoa. The pellet is separated from the supernatant fluid, and some more semen preparation medium is added to the pellet in a test tube and left in the incubator. The active sperms swim up and reach the top layer of the culture medium. After 6 hours, a small drop is examined from the top layer and the number of active sperms is counted. Then 100,000–150,000 (one lac to one and a half lac) sperms are added to each Petri dish containing an egg. These Petri dishes are left in the incubator and examined next morning under

Assisted Reproductive Techniques (Test Tube Baby)

a microscope, for evidence of fertilization, this is visible by the presence of two pronuclei in each egg.

■ LABORATORY PROCEDURES

The laboratory plays an important role in the success of an ART program. A well-equipped laboratory and well-trained embryologist can achieve high success rates. The environment and disposables have to be free of pollution, especially culture medium used for incubation of ova and embryos has to contain correct ingredients for the growing embryos. All the dishes, catheters and test tubes used in the laboratory should be tested for embryo toxicity.

The ova are kept in special incubators, in the culture medium, during their stay outside the human body. Usually after 6 hours of OPU they are reinspected and prepared sperms are added to the dish containing the ova. This is called insemination. Nearly 24 hours later the ova are inspected for fertilization.

After 2–5 days, 2–3 microscopically good looking embryos are loaded in a special catheter for ET.

Endometrial Receptivity Array Test

Many women undergoing IVF are unable to get pregnant, even after transferring good quality embryos. Although a good quality embryo is an important starting point, it is also important to transfer embryo into a uterus that is ready to receive the embryo.

Endometrial receptivity array (ERA) test evaluates endometrial receptivity, the optimal time for ET that is specific for each women.

Endometrial receptivity means when the lining of uterus is ready to receive embryo. It has a success rate of 72% in IVF patients.

■ EMBRYO TRANSFER

The embryos are inspected the subsequent morning for multiplication. After 36–48 hours of OPU, if the embryo is growing well, it should be at 4–6-cell stage.

The embryos are graded as, good, average, and poor according to their appearance. Usually, 1–2 embryos are loaded in a special catheter by an embryologist and then a gynecologist injects these embryos into the uterine cavity through the neck of the womb. This does not cause any discomfort to the patient. She lies on her back for half an hour only. Once the treatment is complete, the patient can go home and pray for success.

■ LUTEAL PHASE SUPPORT

These days almost all patients are advised to use progesterone vaginal tablets, twice a day. The tablets can easily be inserted in the front passage by the patient herself. If a urine or blood test after 14 days of ET shows that pregnancy has taken place, the tablets are continued till 18–20 weeks of pregnancy.

If pregnancy test is negative or the patient gets vaginal bleeding progesterone tablet treatment is discontinued.

■ SUCCESS RATE

In modern times with transfer of technology and international standards of training and standardization, the success rates are comparable in most of the good centers.

Generally, success rates with similar patient data are the same.

In younger patients (<35 years of age), the success rates of achieving pregnancy per OPU are 60–70%. The success rates go down if the wife's age is >40 years.

■ OTHER ADVICE AFTER EMBRYO TRANSFER

Most patients after ET seek advice regarding *rest, diet, exercise, coitus, job, etc.*

I always tell my patients to lead a normal life and carry on with their daily routine. The only precaution is to avoid coitus. Coitus may be avoided during the first trimester (first 3 months of pregnancy). The rest of the factors do not affect the success rate.

There is no need to stay in bed, but do avoid strenuous exercises. There is nothing special about diet. One can eat a normal diet and continue the work as usual. As a matter of fact living normally takes the stress away and may help the pregnancy.

It is important that patients are informed that extra rest or diet do not make any difference to the success rate.

■ PREGNANCY AND TAKE HOME BABY

Once the pregnancy test is positive, it is all celebrations, exchange of greetings, happiness, and joy. There are a few things to remember. ART pregnancy behavior and continuation rates are the same as a spontaneous and natural pregnancy. The risk of complications of pregnancy is the same as after a naturally conceived pregnancy. However, the following risks are more after ART pregnancy:

- *Multiple pregnancies*: In cases where two or three embryos are transferred, the incidence of twins and triplets is nearly 10%. With multiple pregnancies the risk of complications, especially premature birth increases. That is why if there are more than twins, fetal reduction is considered.
- *Early pregnancy loss (miscarriage)*: The risk of miscarriage is slightly higher after ART pregnancy. Miscarriage upsets every patient but after an ART, if miscarriage does takes place, it is definitely more upsetting.
- *Malformation of baby*: The risk of malformation (abnormalities) of a baby after ART is the same as after a spontaneous pregnancy. The incidence of abnormalities among millions of babies born with ART is not higher than the general population.

- *Mode of delivery*: The mode of delivery need not be a cesarean section because of ART. Babies are delivered normally after ART, unless there is a pregnancy complication that requires operative delivery.
- *Take home baby rate*: The take home baby rate is not the same as the pregnancy rate. Due to a higher risk of multiple pregnancies and early pregnancy loss (miscarriage), the take home baby rate is lower than the pregnancy rate. In most of the centers it is 60–70% of overall pregnancy rate.
- *Repeat ART*: In case of unsuccessful ART treatment, some patients decide to make a second attempt immediately. This treatment is extremely stressful, psychologically, emotionally, socially, physically, and of course financially. Generally, it is recommended the next attempt be postponed for 2–3 months. The patient may recover during this period and feel fit to have another attempt. Medically speaking the second attempt at ART can be made immediately after the previous attempt but it is preferable to postpone the next attempt for 2–3 months.

INTRACYTOPLASMIC SPERM INJECTION

This is an improvement in the technology of IVF. The basic treatment, as far as the patient is concerned, is the same as IVF, except that in intracytoplasmic sperm injection (ICSI) technology instead of keeping a female egg with sperms in a dish and allowing natural fertilization over the next 12–24 hours, *one sperm is injected through a needle directly into the female egg*. This technique was initially designed for those couples who had severe oligospermia (low sperm count). Now this technology is used for almost all patients needing ART treatment. It is applicable to obstructive azoospermia, where spermatozoa are procured directly from the testes or proximal part of vas deferens (epididymis). In such a situation, even if a few spermatozoa are procured either by fine needle aspiration or exploration of the testes (PESA/TESA), ICSI is performed and pregnancy can be achieved. In most laboratories, the success rate is comparable with IVF results.

The indications for ICSI are the same as IVF but an additional indication is a previous failed fertilization during IVF treatment.

Preimplantation Cytogenetic Diagnosis (PGD): See Chapter 9.

CRYOPRESERVATION AND FROZEN EMBRYO TRANSFER (FET)

Cryopreservation

- Embryos
- Eggs
- Sperms
- *Embryo cryopreservation*: In IVF/ICSI, if embryos are produced which are more than the required number. Usually, 1–2 embryos are transferred to

avoid risk of multiple pregnancy and ovarian hyperstimulation. The rest of the embryos can be frozen to avoid the need to go through the whole process of IVF/ICSI again. Nowadays embryos cryopreservation is a routine part of IVF/ICSI and it is used to preserve excess number of embryos that are not transferred.

- *Egg freezing*: It is a new technique. It is particularly beneficial for women who may wish to preserve their fertility for future. It offers the chance to preserve eggs for women who are diagnosed with cancer and have to go through treatment such as chemotherapy or radiation which may lead to subfertility.
- *Sperm freezing*: The sperm of man can be frozen due to many reasons, for example, patients with cancers prior to chemotherapy. It is also useful for the couple, if husband is not available at the time of IVF/ICSI.

CHAPTER 8

Treatment of Subfertility (Male Factors)

■ INTRODUCTION

In the male partner, the following defects can be treated by available methods:
- Low sperm count and motility
- Absent sperm in the semen (obstructive azoospermia)
- Impotency.

■ LOW SPERM COUNT (OLIGOSPERMIA)

The first step is to confirm low count or motility by *repeating the test two or three times* over a period of 4-6 months. The parameters for normal semen analysis prescribed by World Health Organization (WHO) are as follows:

The following characteristics of semen are examined:
- Quantity of semen (average 0.2-5 mL)
- *Viscosity*: Normally semen liquefies after half an hour, but if it remains viscous that could be due to infection
- Number of sperms per milliliter (average 20-100 million)
- Motility of the spermatozoa (average 50%)
- Forms or morphology of the spermatozoa (>4% should be normal in shape)
- Presence of pus cells or any other abnormality
- Absence of fructose or acidic pH of semen suggests blockage within the ejaculatory ducts.

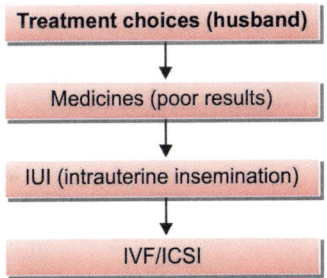

If the count is repeatedly below 20 million/mL then it is considered below the limit prescribed by WHO, but it does not mean that he is not capable of making his wife pregnant. It is quite common to see pregnancies in patients with count and motility below the limit prescribed by WHO. In case the count is low then the couple should be counseled that lower the count lesser are the chances of spontaneous pregnancy.

Treatment of Subfertility (Male Factors)

Unfortunately, there is no identifiable cause in most of these men. There is no special medicine which can help to improve the sperm count. In some men, there may be a minor chromosomal anomaly (microdeletion of chromosome). All treatments prescribed to help the husbands semen quality are empirical. The general advice to these couples is that as long as spermatozoa production is present in the testes, the couple can be helped by any of the modern available methods. The husbands with oligospermia are generally given the following advice:

- The husband is advised not to wear tight under pants and to stop smoking and drinking alcohol
- Cold baths for scrotal area are advisable
- Surgical correction of scrotal abnormality can be carried out (varicocele, hydrocele)
- Improvement of general health
- *Testosterone is not prescribed*. It causes suppression of sperm production, especially if given in large doses for a long period (3-6 months).

About 3-6 months after the treatment described above, semen analysis is carried out to test for improvement. The final decision, in those patients who have persistently low sperm count is a special test in the in vitro fertilization (IVF) laboratory which helps to decide the line of action.

Sperm DNA Fragmentation Test

This test is used to detect sperm DNA damage. This test involves chemically breaking down sperm sample to release the DNA and testing it. A semen sample is needed to perform the test. The result of DNA test aim to indicate the fertility potential of sperm in semen sample. Sperm DNA damage can be associated with subfertility, poor IVF fertilization rates in IVF/ICSI (intracytoplasmic sperm injection).

Sperm Survival Test

For the sperm survival test, the ejaculate is collected and semen is processed as for IVF (test tube baby) treatment. The processed semen is kept in special incubator for 24 hours. After 24 hours, if there are >3 million surviving sperms, then it is assumed that the wife can become pregnant even naturally or by intrauterine insemination (IUI). If after 24 hours the surviving spermatozoa in the specimen are <3 million then the couple needs either IVF or ICSI.

Sperm Deletion Test

Male factor subfertility accounts for almost 50% of the cases presented at IVF clinics. One of the most common causes attributed to this is the absence of genes normally located on a specific region of the long arm of the Y chromosome known as the azospermia factor (AZF) region. These microdeletions result in spermatogenic failure. Y-chromosome microdeletion (YCMD) test is recommended for azoospermic patients to detect these microdeletions. The result of the test provides a prognostic value for the success of testicular sperm retrieval and allows the avoidance of unnecessary invasive procedures on the patient. The test is simply done by means of taking a sample of peripheral blood of the patient.

■ ABSENT GERM CELLS (AZOOSPERMIA)

Absence of germ cells in the semen could be due to:
- Non-production in the testes, atrophy of the testes (gonadotropic atrophy)
- Obstruction in the passages (obstructive azoospermia).

If the cause is *atrophy of the testes*, the response to all types of treatment is poor. The stimulation of testes by drugs has not increased optimism. Such couples need emotional support to face the fact that *no treatment is available*.

Obstruction in the Passages

It can be handled by two methods of treatment:
1. Microsurgical operation
2. Intracytoplasmic sperm injection

Microsurgical Operation

It requires an operating microscope, which is available only in specialized urology centers. The results are not very encouraging. The results depend upon the causative factor and skill of the surgeon. In most of the centers the success rate is between 33 and 66%.

Intracytoplasmic Sperm Injection

This is the latest innovation in IVF technology. Previously for obstructive azoospermia there was no satisfactory treatment. With this technology, in cases of severe oligospermia (very low sperm count or motility), where only a few sperms are available, one sperm is picked up and injected into the egg under a special high-powered microscope with attachment for micromanipulation and microinjection. This has been a real advancement in the treatment of defective semen. In a case of obstructive azoospermia, sperm can be procured by needle aspiration directly from the head of the vas deferens (attachment of male tubes near the testes, epididymis) or directly from tubules of the testes, either by needle aspiration or by surgical biopsy.

This technology provides success rate similar to IVF or in some centers even higher. This process gives real hope to the husbands with a very low sperm count, low motility, and those with obstructive azoospermia.

The details of this treatment are described in Chapter 7.

■ TREATMENT OF UNEXPLAINED SUBFERTILITY

In spite of modern detailed investigations, no fault is found with either partner in more than 10% of the cases. Such couples are declared as cases of *unexplained subfertility*. They feel most frustrated. In spite of going through such elaborate tests and expenses they are still in the dark about their problem. Generally, they get more upset than those in whom some cause has been identified. They need to be reassured, that if they wait a little a longer, there may be a chance of spontaneous conception. "It does happen". Sometimes they conceive during investigations without any treatment, and sometimes immediately after the adoption of a baby.

If a sufficiently long time has elapsed, and a couple insists on some treatment, then the management will be as follows:
- Reassurance (hope, wait, and pray)
- Super ovulation of wife for 2–3 cycles with clomiphene citrate, ultrasound monitoring and timed coitus
- If no luck, IUI for 3–4 cycles
- If still no success, then IVF or ICSI.

In spite of all these treatments, there will be some failures. Then in such cases, the cause could be identified as a *failure of fertilization or implantation* due to either defect in the spermatozoa, which cannot penetrate, or in the shell of the egg which does not allow penetration. Similarly, there could be a defect with the lining of the womb, which does not allow penetration and growth of the fertilized egg (embryo) in the cavity. If any fault is diagnosed, the couple is informed and treated accordingly.

CHAPTER 9

Donor Egg/Sperm and Surrogacy

■ WHAT IS DONOR EGG?

During the treatment of subfertility if egg of another young woman is used to achieve a pregnancy, it is called donor egg pregnancy. Donor egg is the treatment of those subfertile couples in whom the wife for any reason cannot produce an egg. Generally speaking reasons for nonproduction of egg in the wife are:
- Early stoppage of egg production in the ovaries, i.e., premature ovarian insufficiency (POI).
- Age of the wife is near 40 years because of her age production of egg is irregular and imperfect.
- Damage to the ovaries either due to disease or treatment (cancer irradiation)
- When there is repeated failure of stimulation to produce a satisfactory response in the production of eggs.

■ WHAT IS DONOR SPERM?

If during the treatment of subfertility sperm of another man is used to achieve fertilization it is called donor sperm pregnancy. This is the need of those couples where the husband has azoospermia (absence of spermatozoa) in spite of all the treatments. There are no sperms available either in the ejaculate (semen) or directly from the testes. Generally, the reasons for this kind of condition are:
- Husband has genetic problems and the cause of azoospermia is chromosomal or genetic defect.
- Undescended testes, where the testes have remained in the abdomen for a long time and in spite of surgical treatment they cannot produce sperm.
- There is damage to the testes. Either by infection (mumps) or by surgery or irradiation for treatment of cancer.

■ WHAT IS SURROGACY?

If for any medical or social reason, a fertilized egg (embryo) is transferred to the uterus of another woman and it grows insides her uterus for the duration of pregnancy that woman is called the surrogate woman. Surrogacy is the need of those couples where the wife does not have a uterus or pregnancy cannot stay in the uterus because of the defect in the uterus or other social or medical reasons such as:
- Wife cannot carry the pregnancy for medical reasons such as severe heart disease, high blood pressure, and advanced stage of diabetes.

- Absence of the uterus due to diseases such as fibroids or heavy menstrual bleeding.
- *Social reasons*: For professional and social engagements of the wife she cannot afford to carry a pregnancy for 9 months and remain out of job or nonfunctional for a longish period.

We have seen in the last 50 years great developments in medicine and healthcare system. Fortunately during this period, the treatment for subfertile couples has tremendously improved. It is not long ago before the birth of Louise Brown (world's first IVF baby), not much could be done for subfertile couples. The major treatable factors were lower sperm count and difficulty with ovulation. Only few drugs were available to support or enhance their capabilities. In case of blocked tubes not much was available. This was the major factor in South Asian countries responsible for subfertility.

After the birth of baby Brown a new window opened up for such couples. With recent research, the results are going up to nearly 60–70% at most of the ART centers. It shows that we have come a long way but still research is required for those couples who cannot produce eggs or have total absence of spermatozoa. In such cases, current medicine is unable to help.

There are patients who cannot be helped by the available treatment to produce eggs or sperms. In women, this condition may be due to POI or removal of the uterus due to some disease leading to inability to carry a child.

In men, failure to produce sperms may be due to nonobstructive azoospermia. While these patients are desperate to have a baby, the help they require is not accepted universally by certain societies, religions, and countries. This help involves the donation of eggs or sperms from a third party, it is called a donor pregnancy. In cases where the woman cannot carry the baby, a surrogate mother may be involved. Biologically, speaking the baby does not belong to the woman giving birth to the child and he belongs to the woman whose egg was used to form the embryo. In our region, egg/sperm donation or surrogacy is acceptable in countries such as India and Nepal but not in Pakistan, Afghanistan, and Bangladesh.

Such cases where the husband does not produce spermatozoa (sperms) because of nonobstructive azoospermia, donor sperm can help them to have a baby. Such couples face numerous social and religious problems. Biologically, the child belongs to the donor and not to the woman delivering the baby. This kind of third party involvement in the conduct of ART is not universally accepted.

Similarly, the extreme example is when the couple decides for either medical or social reasons that the wife cannot carry the pregnancy for 9 months, such couples may ask for the help of a third party such as a young woman who can carry their embryo for 9 months and give birth to their baby. This baby although remains in the uterus or womb of the third woman it biologically belongs to his/her original parents to whom the egg and sperm belongs. The baby is carried and delivered by another woman who is not the biological mother of the baby. These are complicated situations. Surrogacy is not accepted universally, as a matter of fact most of the countries do not encourage surrogacy but some countries have relaxed rules and regulations on this issue and permit surrogacy with some legal restrictions.

One could object to surrogacy for the reasons of commercialization. Such financial arrangements are to help alleviate misery of desperately needy couples. It is important to remember that there are always social and legal issues in solving human misery. These issues related to surrogacy are present because sometimes the surrogate woman does not wish to part with the baby. She feels she had carried the baby for 9 months. So she feels emotionally attached to the baby. There has to be a legal contract between the surrogate woman and biological parents. It will minimize threats or complications for all the involved parties.

As physicians, we are not directly involved in the financial transactions between the donors and recipients. Similarly, biological parents and surrogate woman must have a legal contract providing protection to the rights of each party. The baby biologically does not belong to the surrogate woman. Legally, ethically and morally the baby belongs to the couple whose egg and sperm were used to produce the embryo but for medical or social reasons the wife had not carried the baby.

There is a large number of couples who are in such situations. Unfortunately, these solutions are not allowed in all countries of our region. We feel those couples who need donor egg and donor sperm or surrogacy they should be at least advised that this kind of technical help is available. They will have to travel to another country or seek assistance somewhere else which is not readily available in their own country. Some countries allow these procedures to promote medical tourism.

There are several medical, ethical, and legal issues related to these situations but we must counsel our patients that if they need this kind of help it may not be available at a particular center. If they are desperate they can seek this help away from that center or the country. The donor egg/sperm and surrogacy have high financial cost which sometimes is too high for the patients. Physicians' responsibility is to provide information to such couples about the possibilities of help.

The matters related to ethical issue are not discussed at length in this chapter. Those who wish to learn in depth may consult larger volumes.

This chapter is included in this book for the couples who decide to have this kind of medical help. They are informed that such medical help is available but not at every ART center.

CHAPTER 10

How to Prepare for a Pregnancy?

■ INTRODUCTION

Once you have decided to have a baby, you must ensure that you are in the best of health. Good health, free of any medical problems means a good pregnancy with fewer risks of complications during pregnancy.

If you are suffering from any medical problems, or taking medicines as a treatment, they might influence the outcome of your pregnancy. It is advisable to consult a doctor before conception so that necessary adjustments are made according to the needs of the pregnancy.

Sometimes one may not be aware of a particular medical problem, *it is suggested that you should have a thorough medical checkup and prepregnancy counseling.*

If your pregnancy is after a prolonged period of subfertility, the following aspects should be considered, before the start of a pregnancy.

■ AGE

The best age to have a baby is between 20 and 25 years. Before the age of 20 years, girl is growing so her body has greater demands for all the nutrient factors. Her reserves of nutrients may not be sufficient to supply the additional needs of a pregnancy. It is a known fact that teenage pregnancy carries higher risks of complications of pregnancy and labor (childbirth).

After the age of 35 years, the stress of pregnancy may cause some medical problems to arise, particularly if there is a family history of such problems. Moreover, certain fetal anomalies such as Down syndrome (mongolism) are more likely to occur after 35 years of age. If you are over 35 years, you will need screening for such problems during your pregnancy.

After the age of 35 years, the fertility of a woman starts declining. If you are already subfertile, the chances of achieving a pregnancy become less. Practically speaking, after the age of 40 years, the chances of pregnancy are extremely low. It is better to complete a family before fertility declines or medical problems, diabetes, hypertension (blood pressure) or any other medical disease arise.

If you got married at an older age and wish to conceive, it is advisable that you seek a medical checkup with all relevant investigations and treatment early, rather than waiting for the customary period of 2 years for a spontaneous pregnancy.

■ WEIGHT

Generally, the average weight in women is 110–150 pounds (see Chapter 5). If you are, either underweight or overweight, you need to consult a doctor because in both situations there is a higher risk of complications during pregnancy.

If you are *underweight* due to a medical disease such as anorexia nervosa, dietary habits or chronic illness they all need to be corrected, otherwise you stand a higher risk of an early miscarriage, small-sized baby, or premature birth of the baby.

If you are *overweight* before the start of a pregnancy (>150 lb), then the risks of deep venous thrombosis (DVT), hypertension, and diabetes are higher during the pregnancy.

A checkup before pregnancy is recommended. In both situations of being under- or overweight, you should try to be of average weight by dietary corrections. If, in addition to weight there are other signs or symptoms of the presence of medical disorders such as polycystic ovaries (PCO) and hirsutism, they require treatment, may be they are responsible for your subfertility or early pregnancy loss.

■ DIET

You need not be on any special diet before you start your pregnancy. If you have been observing certain dietary restrictions you should stop them. If there are special medical reasons, diabetes, hypertension, etc., then you should become even more careful about these restrictions.

Generally, speaking a good comprehensive diet, of vegetables, fruits, and milk products will take care of your needs during pregnancy.

It is recommended that certain supplements of folic acid, calcium, and iron may be added, especially if diet is suspected to be not comprehensive. Folic acid supplement is a useful preventive measure for neural tube defects (spina bifida, etc.) provided it is taken for 3 months prior to pregnancy.

One does not need extra calories, in prepregnancy phase, or even during the first 3 months of pregnancy. Extra green vegetables and a glass of milk will take care of extra needs of iron and calcium. If vegetables and milk are not a part of the daily diet then supplementary tablets may be taken.

■ MEDICAL DISEASES

It is beyond the scope of this book to cover all the medical diseases and their relationship with pregnancy. It is generally recommended that if you have a medical problem, it should be controlled, you should discuss with your doctors the implications of that particular disease during pregnancy. If you are taking any drugs for the treatment of your medical problem, you should know whether that drug can cause any developmental problems to the baby or complications of pregnancy. If such a risk is there, your doctor may change the medication or adjust the dosage. *Most patients need adjustment of dosage of medical drugs during pregnancy.*

The common medical problems that occur during a pregnancy are discussed briefly.

Diabetes Mellitus

Diabetes mellitus has a higher risk of complications during pregnancy. Diabetes affects pregnancy adversely and pregnancy also makes diabetes worse by increasing demands on the dose of insulin.

Generally speaking, oral drugs and hypoglycemic agents used to control diabetes should be reviewed and dosage needs readjustment during pregnancy. It is recommended that diabetic patients should consult a physician before the start of pregnancy.

Diet control should be adjusted according to the needs of pregnancy. If you are not diabetic but you have either a family history of diabetes or any other feature which may indicate that you could develop diabetes later in life, you should be closely watched by repeated blood sugar checks. If at any time the sugar level is high, you may need insulin to control it. Good control of diabetes reduces the risks of complications during pregnancy.

It is important to remember that after pregnancy the diabetic status returns to prepregnancy levels. If you have mild diabetes, and you are on diet control or oral tablets only, you may need insulin during pregnancy. If you need insulin during pregnancy, after the pregnancy is over, you will return to prepregnancy diet and drugs.

Before you embark on a pregnancy you should make sure that your diabetes is well controlled. If you are diabetic then you should take insulin for a better control and also less side effects of the drugs on your baby and pregnancy, particularly during first 3 months of pregnancy.

Hypertension (Blood Pressure)

High blood pressure is quite common in the general population. If you are planning a pregnancy have a checkup of your blood pressure and heart. It is good news if your blood pressure and heart are normal.

High blood pressure should be controlled. There are certain drugs which should not be taken during pregnancy, i.e., angiotensin-converting enzyme (ACE) inhibitors. You should tell your doctor about your future plans of pregnancy, and the drugs should be changed and the dose should be adjusted accordingly.

If you already have blood pressure, it is likely to get worse during pregnancy and create problems with the growth of the baby, preeclampsia and eclampsia (convulsions or fits) and even death of the baby. You require very close monitoring of blood pressure and its complications. Very close monitoring of blood pressure and its complications, good control produces good results.

Certain dietary adjustments, salt restriction and exercise may be useful during pregnancy. *Extra rest is useful but strict bed rest or totally salt free diet is not required.*

Anemia

You may not even be conscious of the fact that you are anemic. This medical disorder is very common in our country. It is either due to poor nutrition or due to chronic blood loss (heavy periods and piles).

Sometimes there are genetically inherited blood diseases which are passed on to the next generation and cause anemia, e.g., thalassemia (major or minor). It is better to have your hemoglobin (Hb) checked and if it is low then it should be investigated and treated accordingly. Oral iron therapy is recommended to treat anemia.

If there is a family history of *thalassemia and you are married to a cousin* then you should seek advice from a blood disease specialist (hematologist) or a geneticist before the start of your pregnancy. You may need investigations during first 3 months of pregnancy—NIPT (noninvasive prenatal testing, Harmony® test), chorionic villus sampling (CVS), by amniocentesis to find out if your baby has inherited this problem.

Systemic Lupus Erythematosus

If you suffer from systemic lupus erythematosus (SLE) or a similar disease, then it is possible that you are on *steroids* or some other drugs. There is a risk of adverse effects of not only the disease but also the drugs on the pregnancy.

Systemic lupus erythematosus carries higher risks of early pregnancy loss (miscarriage) and drugs or steroids may cause certain abnormalities in the baby. You will need special ultrasonographic assessment of the baby at 12th to 14th weeks of pregnancy. You should start your pregnancy, only if your physician is happy with the control of your disease.

Chemotherapy and Cancer

A malignancy in the recent past and radiotherapy or chemotherapy to treat the malignancy *do not preclude a pregnancy.*

Chemotherapy reduces chances of achieving spontaneous, natural pregnancy. Radiotherapy and most of the chemotherapeutic drugs have toxic effects on the ovaries, especially the eggs. It is important that this matter should be discussed with your oncologist who will be able to tell whether your recent disease can be made worse by pregnancy, in this case you should avoid pregnancy (breast cancer). Not all breast cancers are made worse by pregnancy, but your oncologist can advise you correctly.

Similarly, the chemotherapeutic drugs can also cause malformations of the baby or miscarriage. There should be a sufficient gap between the last course of chemotherapy and start of your pregnancy. *Remember, if you had cancer in the past it is not a contraindication for having a baby but clearance from the oncologist is needed.*

Sexually Transmitted Infections

These diseases are passed from one partner to the other during sexual intercourse (coitus).

The following infections are common sexually transmitted infections (STIs):
- *Chlamydia*
- Bacterial vaginosis (BV)
- Gonorrhea
- Herpes
- Syphilis
- Human immunodeficiency virus (HIV) or [acquired immunodeficiency syndrome (AIDS)].

Their presence may cause subfertility due to blockage of the tubes, but not all STIs cause subfertility. Pregnancy can be achieved in the presence of STIs but these diseases may influence the outcome of pregnancy. The disease can be passed on to the baby either during pregnancy or at the time of delivery.

You should have a thorough check up before the start of the pregnancy, ensure that there is no local or general infection. This can be ensured by local tests or blood tests which become positive due to the presence of antibodies (serological tests for antibodies). Generally, pregnancy should be delayed till the disease is treated by appropriate drugs.

■ DRUGS BEFORE THE START OF PREGNANCY

It is better not to take any drugs, for at least 2–3 months prior to the start of pregnancy. *No drug can be declared absolutely safe during pregnancy,* (especially during the first 3 months of pregnancy). Most drugs leave residual traces in the body for a few weeks, even after you have stopped taking them.

When a pregnancy is planned, unless the drug is essential to control a particular disease, one should not take any medication for 2–3 months.

This precaution is particularly important for hormones, antibiotics, chemotherapy, oral hypoglycemic agents, and some of the hypotensive drugs.

If at all, you have to take medication, it should be after consultation with your doctor who should prescribe the safest and best choice for you.

Dosage of certain essential drugs has to be adjusted or sometimes changed according to the needs of pregnancy. Some drugs that control epilepsy are safer than others.

It is better to start some of the vitamins (folic acid) and minerals, which are essential, even before the beginning of pregnancy.

If you are suffering from any of the following diseases, ensure that only those drugs that are safe during pregnancy are taken:
- Psychiatric disorder (depression, anxiety, neurosis, etc.)
- Epilepsy
- High blood pressure
- Diabetes
- Thyroid disease.

All diseases named above may get worse during pregnancy. They need close monitoring and adjustment of the dose of the drugs.
- If you have been on drugs to control polycystic ovarian disease (oral contraceptive pill or other hormones), you should stop taking them for at least 2–3 months before planning the start of the next pregnancy.

Viral Infections and Vaccinations

It is safer and better if there is no viral infection immediately before and during pregnancy.

Some viral infections are more serious than others. Vaccination against such viral infections (rubella, flu, and measles) must be done well before the start of the pregnancy.

It is advisable not to have vaccination with live or attenuated virus (rubella, MMR) during pregnancy. Dead virus, or bacterial and toxoid vaccinations are safe during pregnancy (tetanus toxoid, polio drops).

Travel

Travel is generally safe during early pregnancy but long journey should be avoided or broken into short breaks. This is particularly useful to avoid deep vein thrombosis (DVT).

Job

If you are a working woman, you should continue your job as usual. A change of job is advised only if the present job is physically dangerous or too hectic.

Exercise

You may continue usual exercises and swimming before start of a pregnancy. During pregnancy, it is advisable to carry on with walking and light exercise but one should avoid strenuous workouts.

During pregnancy, walking is generally recommended, the duration may be limited according to your stamina. You should not get tired or exhausted by continuing your exercise unnecessarily for a prolonged period.

Rest

During pregnancy, unless there is a problem, advice is to take life easy. In Pakistan, women are generally over worked (stress of work at job, household chores). In a joint family system the usual social jobs have to be done. It is advisable to rest in the afternoon for a couple of hours. This rest not only improves circulation to the baby but also helps to provide physical rest and relaxation to the woman.

■ COITUS (SEXUAL INTERCOURSE)

Before the onset of a pregnancy there are no restrictions on coitus. During the first 3 months superficial coitus is suggested as this helps in avoiding disturbance of lower part and neck of the womb. Patients who have had a past history of early pregnancy loss or repeated miscarriage may be advised to use condoms. It helps to avoid contact of semen with the neck of the womb (cervix). The semen contains certain chemicals which may initiate uterine contraction and lead to early miscarriage.

■ CLOTHES/SHOES

Generally, women prefer to wear maternity dresses during pregnancy. In our country, ladies clothes (shalwar/kameez) are usually loose fitting. Tight fitting (jeans/blouses) clothes are generally uncomfortable.

Most mothers in law will advise not to wear high heels. I suppose the logic is not to trip while walking. No harm in accepting such friendly advice from a mother-in-law. The objective is to wear comfortable, stable, and loose fitting shoes during pregnancy, because water retention makes the feet swollen in the evening. During pregnancy, avoid long periods of standing or sitting with your feet on the floor. Whenever possible put your feet up on a stool while sitting.

■ FIBROIDS/OVARIAN CYSTS

If an ovarian cyst is diagnosed before the start of the pregnancy, you should have it removed before you become pregnant. On the other hand, if fibroids are diagnosed before pregnancy, during a routine checkup, and are not causing any symptoms, they should be localized by ultrasonography. *If fibroids are not impinging on to the uterine cavity, it is not necessary to remove them before pregnancy.* There is a slightly higher risk of early pregnancy loss or early labor (prematurity), cesarean section, but on the other hand after myomectomy (removal of fibroids), there is a risk of adhesions and tubal blockage leading to subfertility.

If fibroids are not large and not causing symptoms, they may be left on their own. If there is a history of complication of previous pregnancy or fibroids are associated with long subfertility then they may be removed before you embark upon your next pregnancy.

■ FAMILY HISTORY OF ABNORMAL BABIES

Consult a geneticist, he will tell you the percentage of risks of your baby and may suggest tests for the baby, during first 3 months of pregnancy (CVS, ultrasonography, blood hormone tests, NIPT test).

Generally, patients get worried if it is a *marriage between cousins*. Remember that cousin marriage without any family history of babies with abnormality does not carry high risk of abnormality of the baby. In such a case, there is no need to go through elaborate biochemical or invasive tests like CVS. However, you need careful supervision and monitoring because the risks of complications and problems with the baby are still there because of chance happening.

■ SURGERY/OPERATIONS

If you need any kind of surgery or elective operation, it is better to have it done before the start of your pregnancy.

Generally, it is advisable to avoid elective (planned) surgery during the first 3 months of pregnancy. Only emergency surgery (acute appendicitis, etc.) should be carried out during the first 3 months of pregnancy.

■ HEART DISEASE

If you are suffering from any heart disease, you should seek the advice of your heart specialist (cardiologist) to ensure that your heart can stand the stress of pregnancy. During pregnancy, the "work load" of the heart increases two- to threefold. *In spite of all medication and care, there is a high risk that your heart condition will deteriorate during pregnancy*. The congenital heart conditions carry higher risks for the baby because of a short supply of oxygen. If you have had valvular replacement and are on drugs to keep your blood thin (aspirin, anticoagulation drugs), you should ensure that your doctor is comfortable with the type and dosage of the drug you are taking.

It is important to know when to stop taking these drugs before delivery. If you suffer from a heart condition, and are pregnant, you will need close medical supervision, extra rest, avoidance of infections and anemia during pregnancy.

■ SMOKING

Smoking causes higher risks of complications during pregnancy. There is a risk of miscarriage or small size baby intrauterine growth restriction (IUGR).

It is strongly recommended that you give up smoking, a few months before the start of your pregnancy.

■ ALCOHOL/HARD DRUGS

They have an adverse effect on your health and a bad effect on your baby during pregnancy.

They can cause certain malformations of the baby and complications of pregnancy. *It is strongly recommended that you break free from such addictions and be in your best health during pregnancy.*

■ SCREENING FOR HEPATITIS

Hepatitis is endemic in our society. It is important that you should undergo routine screening for hepatitis. If the tests are positive then postpone pregnancy till you have had full medical treatment for the disease. The risks of transmission of hepatitis from mother to the baby are not very high, but it is recommended that you should treat the disease before you become pregnant.

CHAPTER 11: Acceptance of Childlessness and Adoption

■ INTRODUCTION

Recent developments have definitely given a ray of hope to subfertile couples. These days a large number of couples who could not be helped previously are successfully treated. We are lucky that we are living in an age when this type of help is available. Unfortunately knowledge in this field is not complete and the success rate, even in the best centers of the world, is not 100%. I am certain there are large areas of knowledge of physiology, pathology, and anatomy of which we know very little. We have come a long way in acquiring much insight into this complicated problem but we still have to cover large grounds to have fully comprehensive knowledge of this fascinating subject.

In spite of all the optimism there are going to be couples who will be disappointed due to failure of the treatment or nonavailability of any treatment for their problem at this stage.

I suggest to those couples who are not successful in producing a baby to accept this fact that God does not grant everything to everybody. May be He has endowed them with so many other gifts of life, to compensate them for their misfortune.

In spite of modern methods of assistance, couples who fail to achieve a pregnancy go through various phases of emotional upheavals such as:
- Denial
- Depression
- Acceptance

■ DENIAL

In spite of repeated counseling about chances of failure of treatment, most of the patients start their treatment with a positive mind. Even if the success rate is quoted as being very low, they hope that they are going to be successful. When faced with a negative pregnancy result, they just cannot believe it and keep hoping that the result is wrong or the bleeding will settle down with rest and prayer. Sometimes it takes a while for them to come to terms and accept the negative result.

■ DEPRESSION

After acceptance of the result, they all go through depression, the degree of depression varies, depending upon the personality of the couple. Some may recover quickly and be ready to get on with life or may demand another attempt immediately. Others may go into a deep depression and take months to recover or need psychiatric help. Their depression is as if there has been a demise in the family.

▉ ACCEPTANCE

When the phase of acceptance comes in, there could be two possible conclusions:
1. Acceptance of failure but desire to have another attempt at the treatment with donor egg or sperm or surrogacy.
2. Acceptance of childlessness and to live with it.

In case of a desire to repeat the treatment cycle, as described above, the couple should preferably postpone another attempt till they recover almost completely from depression caused by failure of the previous attempt. It may take a few months. Before initiating the next attempt, it should be ensured by clinical and hormonal evaluation that the patient is a good case for ovarian stimulation and risks of ART treatment are minimal including the chances of failure.

A difficult situation arises when the couple has to accept the fact of childlessness and to live with it for rest of their lives. In such a case, there are three options:
1. To go for donor egg and sperm or surrogacy
2. To live and spend the rest of their lives without a child in the family
3. To look for adoption of a baby from within the family, from a hospital, or from an agency which arranges such adoptions.

Life without a Baby

As described in the beginning of this book, there is an inborn desire to have a baby (procreation). A child is needed to carry your name or inherit your property, the desire to have somebody who would take care of you in old age, to have someone as your mirror image to carry your genes, desire to have social and family support, to share your love and care, all this can only be carried out if you can procreate.

To overcome so many desires and to live without a baby is rather difficult, especially, in cases where mother-in-law or family pressures are immense.

In spite of these social, emotional, and family pressures, if a couple decides to live a childless life, they can be counseled about the *positive aspects of such a life*. Imagine a couple living together without any demands and interference by anybody else. It is like early married life when love and care was shared only by the recently married couple. Imagine that period when the couple had all the time in the world to indulge in their hobbies. There is more time to do social work. There is more time and resources available to take care of others' children. One can support young bright nephews and nieces and become a popular uncle or aunt.

ADOPTION

It is not an easy option. Culturally and legally its acceptance is rather limited. *Generally, the family does not welcome this kind of decision.* They may object to adoption, particularly anonymous adoption, on the basis of family traditions and legal implications regarding inheritance, etc.

Once the couple has decided to adopt a baby, then there are two ways of going about it. According to Pakistani culture the easiest way is to adopt a young baby from within the immediate family. Such adoption is generally welcome and accepted by rest of the family. The only disadvantage of such adoption is that when the biological parents are around, they may create emotional and social problems by claiming the child as he grows older or the child himself may decide to go back to his biological parents. This can cause emotional and social problems for the foster parents and the child as well.

The other adoption is of a child, with an unknown background. It is not so easy in our country. If it can be arranged from a large maternity hospital or through an adoption agency, the child will, perhaps, never know his/her biological parents so he is unlikely to go back to the biological parents. For the sake of credibility of the adopted parents, a child should be informed about adoption at an appropriate age, preferably as early as possible.

The difficulty about such an anonymous adoption is not only in arranging it, but also acceptance by rest of the relatives. Sometimes they are opposed to such an adoption, and hostility is shown by the relatives toward the child.

If the couple has managed to adopt a child, then it is the moral responsibility of the couple to provide him/her with the best possible upbringing, grooming, and education. With such an attitude the couple and the child will have a better and stronger bonding with each other.

Remember that treatment of subfertility is stressful and difficult, but raising a child is more difficult, physically, emotionally, socially, and financially. It is a responsibility which one should not accept without giving it a good thought. The desire to have a baby is different, but coping with stress and demands of taking care of a child from infancy to adulthood are greater.

If knowing all the stresses and strains and innumerable difficulties of adoption, one decides to go ahead and adopt a baby then I wish them good luck and hope it is going to bring a lot of joy and happiness to the couple, and their desire of raising a family. Good grooming and education are going to provide a good citizen to the society and serve the country well. I wish you the best of luck in this venture.

LAST WORD: CHILDLESSNESS

If you are a couple who had detailed and thorough investigations and after such a detailed work-up the doctor tells you, even with the latest advanced treatment, you cannot be helped. In spite of your insistence he says there is no help available.

What do you do? Go to another doctor or hospital and ask for help. May be this doctor is not aware of the latest technology. If the answer is the same, what should you do? The other possibility is that you have had certain number of attempts at the suggested treatment without any success. Your doctor may suggest changing the treatment to in vitro fertilization/intracytoplasmic sperm injection (IVF/ICSI) and you have had quite a few attempts at that as well. After all, IVF/ICSI are not only financially exhausting they are emotionally taxing, so you decide "no more" attempts.

If that is the situation and you feel that you are facing a blind alley and feel helpless, you may feel emotionally depressed and have a feeling of an aimless existence.

What do you do? After all you went through investigations and treatment with certain hope. Now you have reached a point of hopelessness.

What should you do? I feel there are certain realities of life which one has to accept as destiny.

After such acceptance one should get on with life. Having children is an important aspect of life but it is not the only objective of living.

There is much more one can do and contribute to one's own progress and add to the welfare of the society.

Instead of running around from one place to another and seeking multiple advices and various treatments, such couples should accept subfertility and plan life without children. They should have a positive approach toward life and contribute wholeheartedly to the welfare of the society. It will indirectly help children of the next generations. At the end, I wish you good luck with your endeavors and a life full of happiness and joy.

Good Luck.

CHAPTER 12

Normal Laboratory Values

■ BLOOD COMPLETE EXAMINATION

Test	Normal range	Unit
Hemoglobin (male)	13.0–18.0	g/dL
Hemoglobin (female)	1.5–16.0	g/dL
Total TBCs	4.00–6.00	10^6/uL
HCT (hematocrit)	36–46	%
MCV	75–95	fL
MCH	26–32	pg
MCHC	30–35	g/d
Platelet count	150–400	10^9/L
MPV	7.5–11.5	fL
WBC (TLC)	4.0–11.0	10^9/L
Neutrophils	40–75	%
Lymphocytes	20–50	%
Monocytes	2–10	%

(MCH: mean corpuscular hemoglobin; MCHC: mean corpuscular hemoglobin concentration; MCV: mean corpuscular volume; MPV: mean platelet volume; WBC: white blood cell)

■ LIVER FUNCTION TESTS

Test	Normal range	Unit
Bilirubin (total)	0.2–1.2	mg/dL
SGPT (ALT)	1–41	U/L
SGOT (AST)	5–40	U/L
Alkaline phosphatase (ALP)	40–129	U/L
Total protein	6.4–8.3	g/dL
Albumin (serum)	3.50–5.20	g/dL
Globulins	2.5–3.5	g/dL
A/G ratio	1.10–2.40	g/dL
Gamma GT	<60	U/L

(A/G: albumin/globulin; ALT: alanine aminotransferase; AST: aspartate aminotransferase; GT: glutamyl transferase; SGOT: serum glutamic oxaloacetic transaminase; SGPT: serum glutamic pyruvic transaminase)

RENAL FUNCTION TESTS

Test	Normal range	Unit
Urea	10–49	mg/dL
Creatinine	0.70–1.20	mg/dL
BUN (blood urea nitrogen)	5.50–23.00	mg/dL
eGFR	>60	mL/min/1.73 m^2

(eGFR: estimated glomerular filtration rate)

SERUM ELECTROLYTES

Test	Normal range	Unit
Sodium	135.0–150.0	mmol/L
Potassium	3.5–5.3	mmol/L
Chloride (serum)	98–112	mmol/L
Bicarbonates (HCO$_3$)	22.0–29.0	mmol/L

LIPID PROFILE

Test	Normal range	Unit
Triglycerides	Up to 150	mg/dL
Cholesterol	50–200	mg/dL
Desirable cholesterol Borderline high cholesterol High cholesterol	<200 200–240 >240	
HDL (cholesterol)	**See below**	**mg/dL**
High risk of CHD Moderate risk for CHD High risk for CHD	<35 35–55 >55	
LDL (cholesterol)	**See below**	**mg/dL**
Optimum level Above optimum level Optimum level Borderline high level High level Very high level	<100 100–129 <100 130–159 160–189 >190	
VLDL (cholesterol)	Up to 25.0	mg/dL
Cholesterol/HDL ratio	3.5–50	

(HDL: high-density lipoprotein; LDL: low-density lipoprotein; VLDL: very-low-density lipoprotein)

Normal Laboratory Values

SPECIAL CHEMISTRY

Luteinizing hormone (LH)	See below	mIU/mL
Follicular phase	2.4–12.6	
Ovulation phase	14.0–95.6	
Luteal phase	1.0–11.4	
Postmenopause	7.7–58.5	
Follicle-stimulating hormone (FSH)	**See below**	**mIU/mL**
Follicular phase	3.5–12.5	
Mid-cycle peak	4.7–21.5	
Luteal phase	1.7–7.7	
Postmenopause	25.8–134.8	
Prolactin	**See below**	**ng/mL**
Male	4.04–15.20	
Female (nonpregnant)	4.79–23.30	
Estradiol (E2)	**See below**	**pg/mL**
Male	7.63–42.6	
Female:		
Follicular phase	12.5–166	
Ovulation phase	85.8–498	
Luteal phase	43.8–211	
Postmenopause	<5.0–54.7	
Pregnancy:		
First trimester	215–4,300	
Children (1–10 years)		
Boys	<5.0–20.7	
Girls	6.0–27.0	
Progesterone	**See below**	**nmol/L**
Female:		
Nonpregnant:		
Follicular phase	0.6–4.7	
Ovulation phase	2.4–9.4	
Luteal phase	5.3–86	
Postmenopausal	0.3–2.5	
Beta hCG (serum)	**See below**	**mIU/mL**
Reference range	<5.30	
After conception		
3 weeks from the last menstrual period	5.30–50	
4 weeks	5.30–426	
5 weeks	19–7,340	
6 weeks	1,080–56,500	
7–8 weeks	7,650–229,000	
9–12 weeks	25,700–288,000	
13–16 weeks	13,300–254,000	
17–24 weeks	4,060–165,400	
25–40 weeks	3,640–117,000	
Postmenopause	<9.5	

Normal Laboratory Values

Test	Normal range	Unit
T3	0.78–2.00	ng/mL
T4	5.56–12.90	µg/dL
Thyroid stimulating hormone (TSH)	0.44–3.63	uIU/mL
First trimester Second trimester Third trimester	0.33–4.59 0.35–4.10 0.21–3.15	
Free T3	See below	pg/mL
Cord Child and adult Pregnancy	1.5–3.91 2.1–4.40 2.0–3.80	
Free T4	See below	pg/mL
First trimester Second and third trimester	0.33–4.59 0.35–4.10	
Total Testosterone	See below	ng/mL

Male (20–49 years):
  >50 years
Female (20–49 years)
  >50 years
	2.49–8.36
	1.93–7.40
	0.084–0.481
	0.029–0.408	

Test	Normal range	Unit
Vitamin B_{12}	223–925	pg/mL
25-hydroxy vitamin-D3 level	See below	ng/mL
Deficiency Insufficiency Sufficiency Potential toxicity	<20 21–29 30–100 >100	
Ferritin	See below	ng/mL
Age group	Reference interval	
Newborn	25.0–200.0	
1 month	200.0–600.0	
2–5 months	50.0–200.0	
6 months	7.0–140.0	

Adults:
  Male
  Female <50 years
  Female >50 years
	
	22.0–350.0
	6.24–140.0
	11.20–264.0	

■ COAGULATION PROFILE

Test	Normal range	Unit
PT (prothrombin)	11.0–14.0	Sec
INR	0.8–1.2	
APTT (activated partial thromboplastin time)	25.0–35.0	Sec
D-dimer	<0.50	µg/mL FEU

■ URINE EXAMINATION REPORT

Physical examination	
Color pale	Yellow
Specific gravity	1.015
Turbidity	Nil
Deposit	Nil
Chemical examination	
pH	6.0
Glucose	Nil
Ketones (urine)	Nil
Protein	Nil
Blood	Nil
Urobilinogen	Normal
Bilirubin	Nil
Nitrite	Negative
Leukocyte esterase	Negative
Microscopy/HPF	
Pus cells	2–3
RBC	Nil
Epithelial cells	Nil
Casts	Nil
Crystals	Nil
Amorphous	Nil

■ SEMEN ANALYSIS

Test	Reference range	Unit
Sample specification		
Sample origin	Sample taken in laboratory	
Days of abstinence	>5 days	
Physical examination		
Volume	2–6	mL
Color	Whitish gray	
Reaction	Alkaline	
Liquefaction	<30	min
Viscosity	Normal	
Sperm count	>15	million/mL
Sperm Motility	>30	
Excellent		%
Good		%
Poor		%
Nonmotile		%
Morphology	>5	
Head piece defects		%
Mid-piece defects		%
Tail piece defects		%
Pus cells	Few	
RBCs	Nil	
Epithelial cells	Nil	

GLOSSARY

Amenorrhea: It means absence of menstruation. If a woman does not bleed at the end of the cycle, this is called amenorrhea. The most common cause of amenorrhea is pregnancy but other diseases may cause amenorrhea.

AMH: This hormone indicates the functioning capacity of the ovaries (ovarian reserve).

Anatomy: Study of the structure of human body

Anovulation: Failure to produce egg. The cause may be in the ovary or in any other part of the body which controls the mechanism of egg production in the ovary.

Apareunia: It is the inability to perform sexual intercourse in the female partner.

Averse to the idea: One opposes a particular thought

Azoospermia: Absence of sperm in the semen

Bartholin's glands: These are small pea-sized glands which are located nearly at the opening of front passage. They create watery secretions to lubricate the front passage during the act of coitus.

Chemotherapy: This is a method to treat the cancer of the body. The treatment is carried out by giving drugs which generally kill the cancer cells.

Chromosomes: These are tiny particles. Their number is fixed for every living organism and for humans. In humans, they are 46 in number. They are paired, so 46 make 23 pairs. One pair is responsible for sex of the baby. This pair is labeled as X and Y. In females, this pair is XX and in male it is XY.

Cilia: The tiny hair-like structures lining the tubes of the womb. Their movements are essential for pushing the early egg or embryo toward the cavity of the womb.

Coitus: It is the sexual act. Male and female indulge in this act. Male partner manages to deposit semen high up into the front passage of the female. Ejaculate contains the sperms which are motile and responsible for fertilization and pregnancy.

Congenital: The child is born with a defect which had developed during the growth of the baby inside mother's womb. This may also result in early childhood diseases. These diseases may be inherited by chromosomal defects or genetic mutation.

Contraindications: Certain treatments cannot be given to the patient because there is risk of abnormal response of the patient.

Glossary

Corpus luteum: This is the part of the follicle or the area from where the egg is released. After the release of the egg, the part of the follicle is called corpus luteum. It continues to function and produce hormones. It is slightly yellowish in color. Two hormones, called estrogen and progesterone, are produced by corpus luteum.

Counseling: The treating doctor explains to the patient various aspects of her problem and management. This is the most important component of management of any patient.

Cryopreservation: This method of preservation is used to store egg, sperm, and early embryo at a very low temperature. This method of preservation is used for later or future use of egg, sperm, and embryo in ART.

Cycle: The menstrual cycle of the female. It generally lasts for 21–35 days. At the end of the cycle every month, bleeding takes place for 4–5 days.

Cyclical fashion: The changes which take place regularly after a certain period.

Dyspareunia: Painful intercourse

Ejaculate (semen): It consists of the secretions produced and stored in the male genital system. These secretions are thrown out at the peak of sexual act as semen or ejaculate. It contains male germs and other secretions produced by the glands close to the genital tract.

Embryo transfer (ET): During ART treatment embryo/embryos grown in the laboratory are transferred into the uterus. Usually only one embryo is inserted into the uterus and this is called SET (single embryo transfer).

Endometrium: It is the lining of the womb. It changes in thickness during each menstrual cycle. It produces secretions to receive the fertilized egg. It provides nourishment to the egg. The fertilized egg implants in the endometrium for further growth of the embryo.

Erectile tissue: Erectile tissue is a part of the male sexual organ. When it is congested, the blood accumulates in that part of the body. It is responsible for stiffening and lengthening of the male organ or penis.

External organs: Those parts which are present outside of the human body.

Fertilization: Union of sperm and egg in the human body, which leads to creation of new being.

Fibroids: This is a tumor-like growth which takes place in the uterus or the womb. Fibroids are benign tumors they rarely become malignant. They could be small in number or large in size and they are responsible for enlargement of the uterus.

Fine needle aspiration cytology (FNAC): This test is used to find out sperm production in the testis. This is a useful test which is usually carried out on those men who have absence of sperm in the semen (azoospermia).

Fetus: This terminology is used for the early growing human being inside the womb (uterus).

Follicle: Follicle is the tiny cyst type formation in the ovary. It is responsible for production of eggs. In this small cyst, there is fluid and an egg. We can observe growth of a follicle in the ultrasound scan (USS). This helps us to know how the egg is progressing or maturing.

Follicle-stimulating hormone (FSH) and luteinizing hormone (LH): These two hormones are secretions which are produced by a small tiny pea-sized organ located at the base of the brain called pituitary. FSH and LH are responsible for the growth of the egg and production of hormones of the ovary and testes.

Genital organs: The parts of the body which are responsible for reproduction.

Gonadotropin-releasing hormone (GnRH) analogs/antagonists: GnRH analogs or antagonists are drugs which have either similar action like gonadotropins or they stop action of the gonadotropins. These drugs are used for stimulation of the ovary to produce more eggs during the treatment of subfertility.

Gonadotropins: These hormones are responsible for stimulation of the ovary to produce egg. These hormones can be given in the form of injections to achieve the same results during ART treatment.

Hernia: Hernia is the weakness in the abdominal wall through which the intestines protrude when the person increases the pressure inside the abdomen by coughing and sneezing.

Hormone/testosterone: Hormones are secretions in the body which are responsible for performance of various functions of the body, i.e., like testosterone is responsible for various functions of the male body. They express male characteristics physically, i.e., growth of beard and other body changes. They are responsible for the male sexual functions.

HSG (X-rays of the tube): X-rays of the tubes is also called hysterosalpingogram. This test is used to find out whether tubes are open or not. It requires injection into the uterus and tubes then X-rays are taken which outline the uterus and tubes and spillage inside the abdomen.

Hydrocele: Accumulation of fluid around the testis in the scrotum.

ICSI: Intracytoplasmic sperm injection (ICSI) is the method where a sperm is injected directly into the egg under microscope. This ensures fertilization. This is part of in vitro fertilization (IVF)

Implantation: This is embedding of the fertilized egg into the lining of the uterus. It takes place 3–4 days after fertilization. The fertilized egg grows and gets attached to the lining through the development of placenta.

Impotence: This is the weakness on the part of male partner which leads to inability to perform intercourse (coitus). The man cannot perform the act of intercourse due to this weakness. This may be due to psychological cause or local physical factor.

Impotency or frigidity: Impotency is the problem with the male where he is unable to achieve erection of his penis for sexual act. Frigidity is the problem with the female partner where she is unable to relax and let the male partner insert his male organ or penis into the front passage of her vagina.

Induction of ovulation: Stimulation of the ovaries by drugs to produce eggs for the treatment of subfertility.

Inheritance: Something one gets from his parents. It may be characteristics, features or property. Inheritance is transfer of those features or property to the next generation.

Instinctive desire: Inner desire or wish to perform

Internal organs: Those parts which are present inside the human body.

Intrauterine insemination (IUI): This is the method of insertion of processed sperms into the uterine cavity. This improves the chances of achieving a pregnancy. This is the most popular method used to assist patients with unexplained subfertility.

Introitus: Opening of the front passage of the female to the outside.

IVF: In vitro fertilization (IVF) means fertilization of the egg takes place outside the human body. In ART, it takes place inside a dish in the laboratory.

Karyotyping: This is a study of body cells for the presence of number of chromosomes. Every human being has 46 chromosomes. They are in the form of 23 pairs. This test shows the presence of number of chromosomes and their normality.

Lactation: Lactation is breastfeeding of the baby.

Laparoscopy: This is a procedure in which an instrument is inserted into the abdomen through a small hole. The instrument is connected to a telescopic system. The operator is able to see inside the abdomen. Generally, this method is used to look at the uterus, tubes, and ovaries in the abdomen. This helps to find out if there is any abnormality. It gives visual information about the presence of any disease or abnormality of the uterus and tubes. This method can also be used to perform surgery.

Leukorrhea: Excessive production of normal secretions in the vagina. Generally, these secretions are colorless odorless and nonirritant.

Leydig cells: Leydig cells are special cells present in the testis. They are responsible for the production of hormones and they do not have direct connection with the production of male germs or sperms. Even if the production of male sperms stops. Leydig cells continue to produce the hormones, i.e., testosterone.

Libido: Desire to have sex, it is variable among human beings.

Luteal phase support: That period of treatment in ART in which after transfer of embryo into the uterus, certain medicines are given for 2–3 months to support implantation and growth of the embryo inside the uterus.

Male hormones: Testosterone is male hormone which is responsible for various male features, i.e., beard, muscular growth, and sexual function.

Malformation: Abnormal formation of any part of the body during development inside the womb of the mother.

Menopause: Menopause is the age at which a woman stops menstruating. It is usually between 45 and 50 years of age. Along with stoppage of menstruation other changes in the body lead to nonproduction of the eggs and degenerative changes or aging changes in the body.

Menstruation: It is the bleeding which takes place during menstrual cycle. Usually, it is about 80–100 mL each month.

This bleeding is due to shedding of the lining of the womb and this happens because of withdrawal of various secretions (hormones) in the body.

Metabolic disease: These diseases are related to the functioning of the body and they are related to production and utilization of sugar, proteins, and fats. Diabetes is related to the production and utilization of sugar. Jaundice is the condition when various secretions produced in the liver accumulate in the body and lead to yellow discoloration of the skin.

Miscarriage: Loss of pregnancy during first 5 months. During this period, the baby is considered not viable. World Health Organization (WHO) has defined viability as a period of 24 weeks of pregnancy.

Monitoring: Close supervision to see the response of the patient to the drugs which are given for certain treatment or stimulation of the ovaries to produce more eggs. Monitoring is carried out personally by observations and by performing certain tests.

Motile: It means moving. This is the normal quality of active male germs.

Motility: Movement of the male germ cells. This movement is responsible for the germ cells to reach the egg in the female.

Multiple pregnancy: There is more than one baby growing inside the uterus, it is called multiple pregnancy. Most commonly, it is twins but sometimes there could be three or four babies simultaneously growing inside the uterus.

Mumps: This is infection of the salivary glands. These glands produce secretions in the mouth called saliva. This infection is caused by a virus. In some cases, this infection also damages testis and ovaries.

Nonobstructive azoospermia: Sperms are not being produced in the testis. The defect could be in the testes or in the production of hormones which control the functions of testes.

Numerical superiority: The numbers are greater than others. There is superiority in numbers.

Obstructive azoospermia: There is some obstruction in the small tubes which carry sperms from testis to the storage place. In this case, the sperms are being produced in the testis normally but they cannot reach the storage place (seminal vesicles). The sperms are absent in the semen but they are present in the testis.

Oligospermia: The sperms are present in the semen but their count is lesser than the prescribed limit of WHO (World Health Organization).

Organs: Various parts of the human body which perform different functions.

Orgasm: This is the height of excitement during sexual act which is achieved by the male or female partner. It is generally achieved by both but timing could be different for each partner. It may not always be achieved during the sexual act. Sometimes the female partner may not achieve orgasm as the male partner gets it more frequently.

Ovarian stimulation: It is part of the treatment of subfertile couples. Medicines are given to stimulate the ovaries to produce more eggs, it is the basic need for the treatment of ART.

Ovulation: The production of an egg and its release from the ovary. It usually happens in the middle of menstrual cycle of the woman. Once the egg is released, it is viable only for 24 hours. If it is not fertilized, it undergoes degeneration.

PCO (polycystic ovaries): In this condition, there are multiple small cysts in the ovary and ovulation is infrequent. It is a common disease among Asian women.

Peristalsis: These are involuntary movements which take place inside the human body. They are always present in the intestine. These movements also take place in the tubes of the female womb. These movements push the female egg toward the cavity of the womb.

PGT: Preimplantation genetic testing (PGT) is used for testing of embryo for any abnormal chromosomes or genetic disease. This is the latest development in the treatment of ART for subfertile couples.

Physiology: Study of the various functions of human body.

PID: Pelvic inflammatory disease. It is infection in the genital tract, i.e., in the uterus, tubes and ovaries.

Placenta: It is the part which gets attached to the lining of the womb. It provides nourishment to the growing baby inside the cavity of the womb.

Procedures of ART: The methods used for treatment of subfertility. After identifying the cause/reason for subfertility, the couple is given treatment accordingly. Generally, IUI, IVF, or ICSI are the methods which are in use.

Procreate: To achieve pregnancy and produce children.

Progesterone: This hormone is produced only when there is production of egg. Estrogen is continuously produced in the body even when there is no production of egg.

Prolapse: It is the weakness of the supports of uterus. Due to this weakness the womb slides downward. It leads to the displacement of the uterus and front passage.

Prostate gland: It is a small organ in men. It is located under the urinary bladder.

Protocols of stimulation: These are the plans or steps laid down for use during stimulation of the ovaries for production of extra eggs. The plans are different for each drug and patient.

Psychological disease: Disease related to functions of the brain.

Puberty: It is the age of a person when rapid growth of various parts of the body takes place and usually it happens between 12 and 18 years of age.

Quacks: Those persons who are practicing medicine but they are not qualified to practice, they are not trained to dispense any medical treatment. This activity is not allowed legally.

Reproduce, reproduction: Produce something which is similar to previous production.

Glossary

Secondary sexual characters: Those features of the body which develop in women and men differently. The presence of such features and their development shows normal functioning of the hormones inside the human body.

Secretions: Secretions are watery productions of various glands. Their quantity and consistency are variable.

Semen: Semen consists of the secretions which are passed out by the male into the front passage of the female partner during sexual intercourse.

Single embryo transfer (SET): When single embryo is transferred into the uterus during the treatment of ART, it is called SET.

Sperm count: Number of sperms in the semen, generally we count them in millions per milliliter.

Sperm motility: Sperms are capable of moving on their own and generally they move fast forward.

Spermatogenesis: Production of sperms in the testis.

Spermatozoa/germ cells: Germ cells are tiny moving particles in the semen. They are responsible for fertilization and pregnancy.

STIs: Sexually transmitted infections. These infections are passed from one partner to the other partner during sexual intercourse.

Subfertility: A couple living together trying to achieve a pregnancy but fails. In young couples, the period may be 2 years and those who are in the late 30s it is 1 year.

Testosterone: Testosterone is the secretion produced by male testis. This is the hormone which is responsible for the growth of hair, beard, and other male characteristics. These hormones are produced by small cells called Leydig cells in the male organs called testis.

Trophoblast: It is the early covering of the fertilized egg or embryo which is essential for its protection and also implantation into the lining of the womb.

Unexplained subfertility: A couple is diagnosed as a case of unexplained subfertility if they had all the available investigations but the doctors are unable to find the cause of failure to achieve pregnancy. The doctors are unsuccessful to pinpoint the cause of subfertility. A large number of couples belong to this group, however most of them can be helped by modern techniques of ART.

Vaginismus: When the female partner does not relax and allow sexual intercourse due to some fear or phobia for this kind of action.

Varicocele: Dilatation of blood vessels around the testis in the scrotum

Vasectomy: This operation is performed on the narrow tubes of a man. The tubes carry sperms from the testis to the storage place (seminal vesicles). During vasectomy, the tubes are cut to ensure that sperms cannot reach the storage place, hence during sexual intercourse no sperms are present in the semen. This method is used for family planning. In such cases, the male partner is responsible for family planning.

X-ray/irradiation: These are the invisible rays which are produced by special machines and they attack the living cells in the body and destroy them. X-ray is also used in small doses to find out shadows inside the body. This is the diagnostic use of X-rays.

Index

Page numbers followed by *f* refer to figure, *fc* refer to flowchart

A
Acquired immunodeficiency syndrome 62
Activated partial thromboplastin time 75
Adoption 69
Advice regarding hygiene 33
Alanine aminotransferase 71
Albumin 71
Alcohol 66
Alkaline phosphatase 71
Amenorrhea 18, 19, 35, 77
American Society of Reproductive Medicine 31
Anemia 61
    correction of 33
Angiotensin-converting enzyme inhibitors 60
Anovulation 77
Antagonist protocol 45
Anti-Mullerian hormone 34
Antral follicle count 30, 34
Anus 6
Anxiety 63
Apareunia 20, 77
Aromatase inhibitors 34, 35
Aspartate aminotransferase 71
Assisted reproductive technique 32, 36, 38, 39, 43, 44
    procedures of 83
    stages of 44
Asthenospermia 16
Azoospermia 4, 16, 18, 22, 24, 41, 53, 77, 79
    factor region 52
    nonobstructive 82
    obstructive 44, 51, 82

B
Bacterial vaginosis 19, 62
Bartholin's glands 6, 77
Basal body temperature chart 26
Beta-human chorionic gonadotropin 73
Bicarbonates 72
Bilirubin 71
Blood
    complete examination 71
    pressure 58, 60
        high 60, 63
    urea nitrogen 72
Body mass index 30, 39
Borderline high cholesterol 72
Brain 13

C
Cancer 61
    irradiation 55
Cervical mucus
    hostility 39
    self-test of 26

Cervix 7, 13, 26
Chemotherapy 17, 61, 77
Chlamydia 19, 62
Chloride 72
Cholesterol 72
    high 72
Chorionic villus sampling 61
Chromosomal defects 16
Chromosome 77
    studies of 24
Cilia 14, 77
Clomiphene 35, 36
    citrate 33-35, 38
Coagulation profile 75
Coital difficulties 22
Coitus 6, 7, 10, 13, 64, 77
    infrequent 20
Controlled ovarian stimulation 38, 44
Convulsions 60
Cornual block 29*f*
Corpus luteum 78
Creatinine 72
Cryopreservation 49, 78
    bank 17
Cyclical fashion 78

D
Deep vein thrombosis 59, 63
Delivery, mode of 49
Depression 63, 67
Diabetes mellitus 58-60, 63
Diet 59
Donor
    egg 55
    sperm 55
        pregnancy 55
Down's syndrome 58
Ducts 3, 5
Dyspareunia 78

E
Eclampsia 60
Eggs 49
    fertilization of 10, 11
    freezing 50
    retrieval of 44
Ejaculation 4, 78
    premature 20, 22, 40
Embryo 14, 43, 49, 54, 55
    cryopreservation 49
    transfer 32, 43, 44, 47, 48, 78
Endometrial biopsy 27
Endometrial receptivity array test 47
Endometriosis 19, 44
Endometrium 7, 78
Epididymis 5

Epilepsy 63
Epithelial cells 76
Erectile dysfunction 20, 22
Erectile tissue 4, 78
Estimated glomerular filtration rate 72
Estradiol 73
    hormonal estimation of 26
Estrogens 8, 9, 12
European Society of Human Reproduction and Embryology) 31
Exercise 63

F

Fallopian tubes 6, 8, 13, 14, 30
Fatigue 35
Female eggs 10, 12
    cell 10
    defect in production of 18
    production of 8, 25
Female front passage 6
Fertilization 8, 10, 11, 13, 43, 44, 78
    failure of 54
Fertilized egg, embedding of 10
Fetus 10, 79
Fibroids 19, 30, 64, 78
Fimbrial block 29f
Fine-needle aspiration cytology 24, 79
Fits 60
Flu 63
Follicle-stimulating hormone 11, 24, 33-35, 73, 79
Frigidity 13, 80
Frozen embryo transfer 38, 49
Fructose, absence of 24, 51

G

Genital organs 3, 79
    female 6, 6f, 7f, 10
    male 3, 3f, 5, 6, 10
Genital tract, congenital defects of 39
Germ cells 5, 84
    absent of 53
    male 10, 11, 16
Globulin 71
Glutamyl transferase 71
Gonadotropin 34, 36, 46, 79
    preparations 37
    releasing hormone 35
        analogs 79
        antagonists 79
Gonads
    female 6, 8
    male 4
Gonorrhea 22, 62

H

Hair, excessive growth of 21
Hard drugs 66
Head piece defects 76
Headache 35
Heart disease 65

Heat flash 36
Heavy periods 61
Hemoglobin 61, 71
Hepatitis 66
    screening for 66
Hernia 79
    operation for 21
Herpes 62
Hormone 5, 79
    female 8
    male 10, 11, 81
    profile 24, 27
Hot climate 17
Human body, structure of 77
Human cell, normal 11
Human chorionic gonadotropin 35
Human immunodeficiency virus 62
Husband's low count 44
Husband's test 23f
Hydrocele 4, 17, 23, 79
Hydrosalpinx 29
Hymen 7
Hypertension 58-60
Hypospadias 8, 40
Hysterosalpingography 28, 34, 39

I

Implantation 10, 14, 44, 54, 80
Impotence 13, 16, 18, 51, 80
In vitro fertilization 17, 27, 32, 43, 52, 70, 79, 80
Infections 17-19, 34, 39
Injury 17
Insemination 44
Instinctive desire 00
Intestinal tract 6
Intracytoplasmic sperm injection 17, 32, 49, 53, 70, 79
Intrauterine growth restriction 65
Intrauterine insemination 40, 80
    indications for 40
    repeated failure of 44
Intrauterine sperm injection 41, 42
Introitus 80
Irradiation 85

K

Karyotyping 24
Klinefelter syndrome 16

L

Lactation 18, 80
Laparoscopic ovarian diathermy 34, 38
Laparoscopy 28, 30, 80
Letrozole 34, 35
Leukorrhea 81
Leydig cells 12, 81, 84
Libido 5, 22, 81
Lipid profile 72
Lipoprotein
    high-density 72
    low-density 72
    very-low-density 72

Index

Liver function tests 71
Low sperm count 51
Luteal phase support 44, 47, 81
Luteinizing hormone 11, 24, 26, 33, 35, 73, 79
Lymphocytes 71

M

Malformation 81
Maturation 12
Measles 63
Menopause 8, 81
Menstrual cycle 30
Menstruation 8, 19, 81
    absence of 18
    heavy 21
    irregular 21
Metabolic disease 81
Metformin 34
Microsurgical operation 53
Mid-cycle peak 73
Mid-piece defects 76
Miscarriages 48, 81
    history of 21
Misconceptions 4
Monocytes 71
Monopolar diathermy 38
Mood swings 35
Motility 82
Multiple births 37
Mumps 17, 22, 55, 82
Muscle aches 35

N

Nausea 35
Nervous system 13
Neurosis 63
Neutrophils 71
Noninvasive prenatal testing 61

O

Oligospermia 4, 16, 41, 44, 51, 82
Oral contraceptive pill 63
Organs 82
    external 78
    function of 3
    internal 80
    male 3
    structure of 3
Orgasm 82
Ova 10, 12
Ovarian cysts 64
Ovarian hyperstimulation syndrome 37
Ovarian stimulation 40, 41, 45, 82
Ovaries 6, 8, 30, 55
    controlled stimulation of 33, 44
    hyperstimulation of 36
    monitoring of 44
    overstimulation of 37
    stimulation of 37
Overweight 21
Ovulation 12, 18, 82
    absent of 34fc, 44
    induction of 32, 33, 80
    infrequent 44
    phase 73
    predictor kit 26
    tests of 25
Ovum 8, 10, 12
    pick up 44, 46

P

Painful sexual intercourse 20
Passages, obstruction in 16, 18, 19, 53
Pelvic inflammatory disease 83
Pelvic organs 21
Penis 3, 4
    malformation of 18
Periods 8, 12
Peristalsis 14, 83
Phallus 3
Piles 61
Pipelle test 27
Pituitary gland 11
Placenta 83
Platelet count 71
Polio drops 63
Polycystic ovarian
    disease 38, 63
    syndrome 33, 34, 38
Postcoital test 34
Potassium 72
Preeclampsia 60
Pregnancy 1, 3, 5, 10, 48, 58, 73, 65
    establishment of 14
    loss, early 48
    multiple 36, 48, 82
    spontaneous 58
Preimplantation genetic testing 83
Premature ovarian insufficiency 55
Progesterone 8, 9, 12, 25, 73, 83
    test 27
Prolactin 24, 73
Prolapse 39, 83
Prostate gland 5, 83
Prostatitis 21
Prothrombin 75
Psychiatric disorder 63
Psychological disease 83
Puberty 8, 83
Pus cells 76
    presence of 24, 51

Q

Quacks 83

R

Renal function tests 72
Reproduction 3, 83
    organs of 4
Royal College of Obstetrics and
    Gynaecology 31
Rubella 63

S

Saline infused sonography 34
Scrotum 3, 4
    local diseases of 17
Secretions 84
    production of 5
Semen 18, 51, 78, 84
    absent sperm in 51
    acidic pH of 24, 51
    analysis 23, 39, 52, 76
    failure to deposit 16, 18
    preparation 44, 46
    quantity of 24, 51
Seminal vesicles 5, 85
Serum glutamic oxaloacetic transaminase 71
Serum glutamic pyruvic transaminase 71
Sex 13
Sexual intercourse 10, 13, 20, 64
Sexually transmitted infections 19, 21, 62, 84
Single embryo transfer 84
Sodium 72
Sonohysterography 28
Sperm 10, 11, 49
    count 4, 76, 84
    defect in production of 16
    deletion test 52
    DNA fragmentation test 52
    freezing 50
    motility 4, 84
    per millilitre, number of 24, 51
    production 5, 10, 17
        suppression of 17
    survival test 24, 52
Spermatogenesis 16, 84
Spermatozoa 5, 10, 11, 13, 16, 18, 19, 84
    absence of 24, 55
    morphology of 51
    motility of 24, 51
    shapes of 24
Stimulation
    monitoring of 46
    protocols of 38, 83
Subfertility 16, 19, 21, 33, 33*fc*, 39, 84
    causes of 16, 18
    investigations of 21
    primary 21
    treatment of 32, 51, 55
    unexplained 16, 32, 40, 44, 54, 84
Surgery 17, 18, 32, 65
Surrogacy 55, 57
Swelling, local 21
Syphilis 17, 62
Systemic lupus erythematosus 61

T

Tail piece defects 76
Test tube baby 43
    treatment 27
Testes 3, 4
    atrophy of 53
    biopsy of 24
    hormones 24
    tumors of 17
Testosterone 5, 12, 24, 52, 79, 84
    hormone 11, 12
Tetanus toxoid 63
Thalassemia 61
Thyroid
    disease 63
    function tests 24
    peroxidase 34
    stimulating hormone 24, 34, 74
Total protein 71
Total testosterone 74
Toxoid vaccinations 63
Transvaginal sonography 26, 46
Triglycerides 72
Trophoblast 84
Tubal insufflation test 28
Tubal ligation, bilateral 39
Tube, X-rays of 24, 79
Tuberculosis 17-19, 22
Tumors 17, 19

U

Ultrasonography 26
Ultrasound 26
    scan 79
Undescended testes 17
Urea 72
Urethra 4, 6
Urethritis 21
Urinary human menopausal gonadotropins 37
Uterus 6, 7, 30
    fallopian tubes of 13

V

Vagina 6, 7, 16, 18, 43
    hostility of 32
Vaginal ultrasound 36
Vaginismus 18, 20, 84
Varicocele 4, 17, 23, 84
Vas deferens 5, 16, 18
Vasectomy 85
Viral infections 63
Viscosity 24, 51, 76
Vision, blurring of 35
Vitamin B12 74
Vomiting 35
Vulva 6

W

Weight 39, 59
White vaginal discharge 7
Womb 6, 7
    biopsy of lining of 27
World Health Organization 51, 81

X

X-rays 17, 24, 28, 79, 85

Y

Y-chromosome microdeletion test 53